understanding

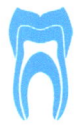

TEETH

An Illustrated Overview of Dental Concepts

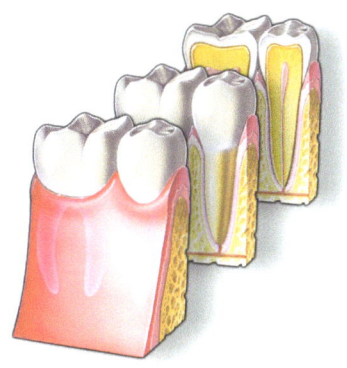

Deluxe Edition

Created and illustrated by:
Stephen F. Gordon, B.A.

Acknowledgement: David M. Niesslein, D.M.D.

dedicated to
Terri

The content herein is provided only as a general overview of some modern dental concepts, and is not intended for, nor to be used as a replacement for individual oral and dental care under the supervision of a qualified dental professional.

Published by Stephen F. Gordon

www.sgordon.com

Contents

Normal Teeth

The health of ones teeth is very important to proper digestion of food and ones overall health. Teeth are living structures with a complex system of support.

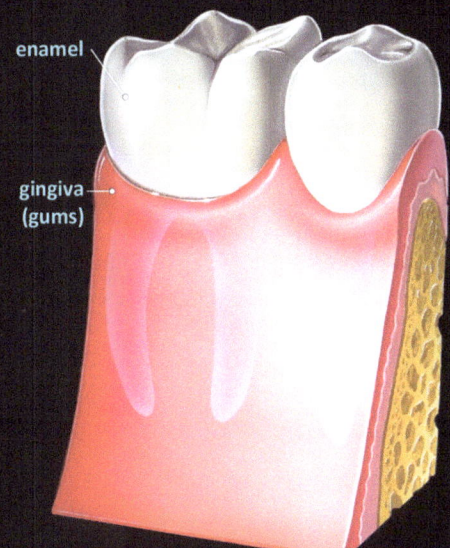

enamel

gingiva (gums)

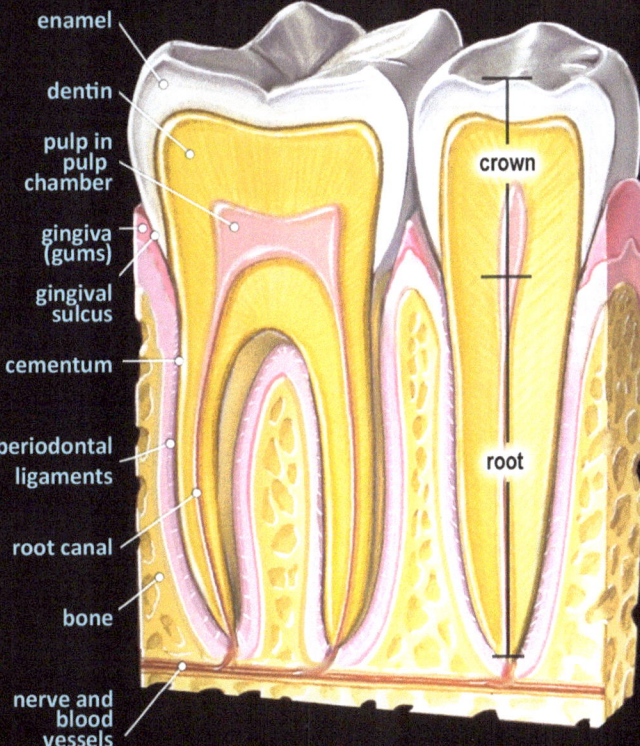

enamel

dentin

pulp in pulp chamber

gingiva (gums)

gingival sulcus

cementum

periodontal ligaments

root canal

bone

nerve and blood vessels

crown

root

1

Primary Teeth

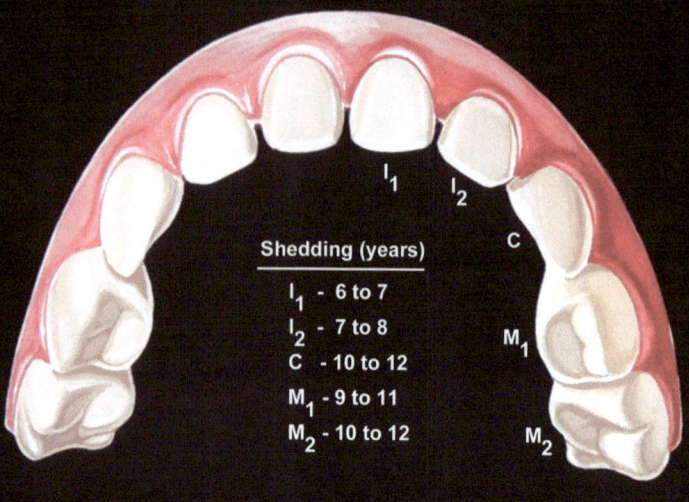

Shedding (years)

I_1 - 6 to 7
I_2 - 7 to 8
C - 10 to 12
M_1 - 9 to 11
M_2 - 10 to 12

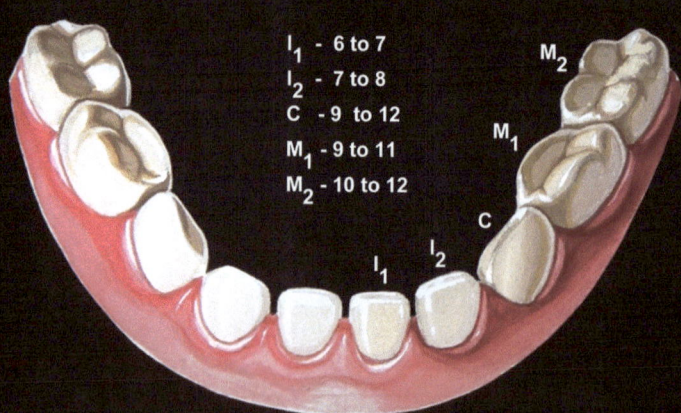

I_1 - 6 to 7
I_2 - 7 to 8
C - 9 to 12
M_1 - 9 to 11
M_2 - 10 to 12

The set of primary teeth typically consists of 20 teeth, and the eruption and shedding times may vary.
I - incisors C - canines M - molars

Permanent Teeth

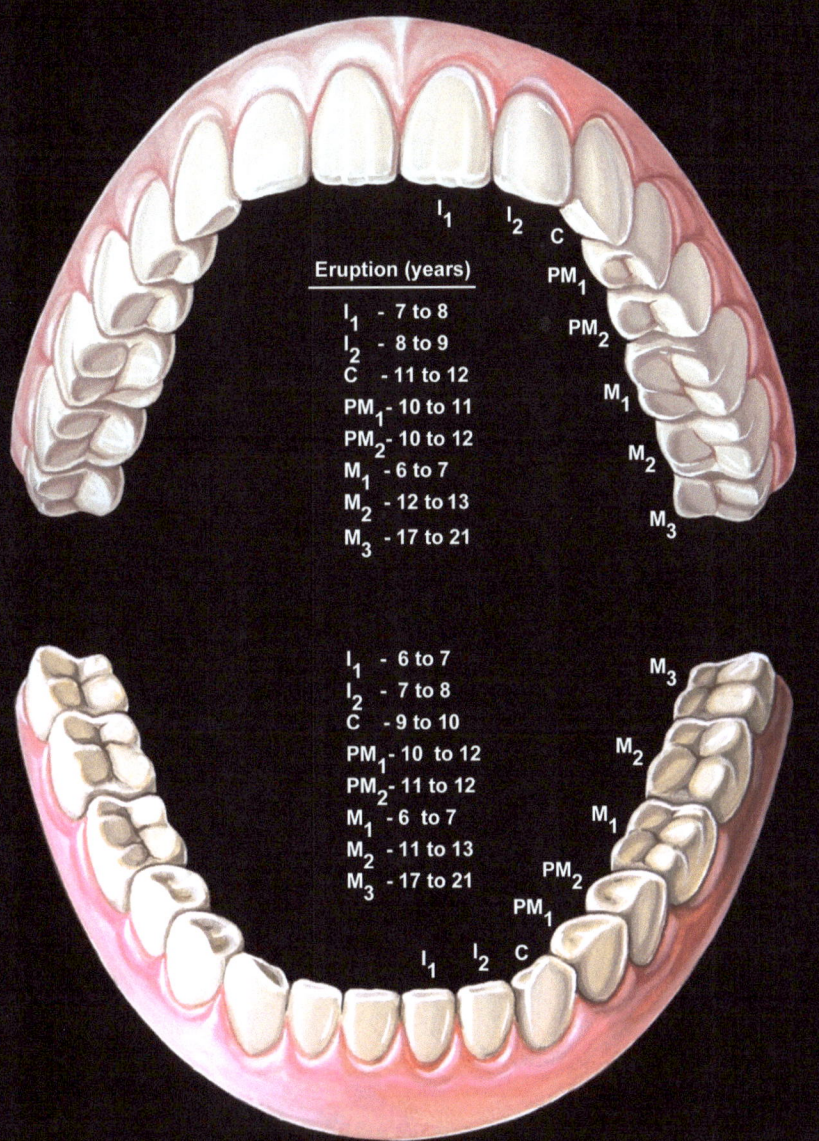

Eruption (years)

I_1 - 7 to 8
I_2 - 8 to 9
C - 11 to 12
PM_1 - 10 to 11
PM_2 - 10 to 12
M_1 - 6 to 7
M_2 - 12 to 13
M_3 - 17 to 21

I_1 - 6 to 7
I_2 - 7 to 8
C - 9 to 10
PM_1 - 10 to 12
PM_2 - 11 to 12
M_1 - 6 to 7
M_2 - 11 to 13
M_3 - 17 to 21

The set of permanent teeth typically consists of 32, and the eruption times may vary.
I - incisors C - canines PM - premolars M - molars

3

Tooth Decay & Repair

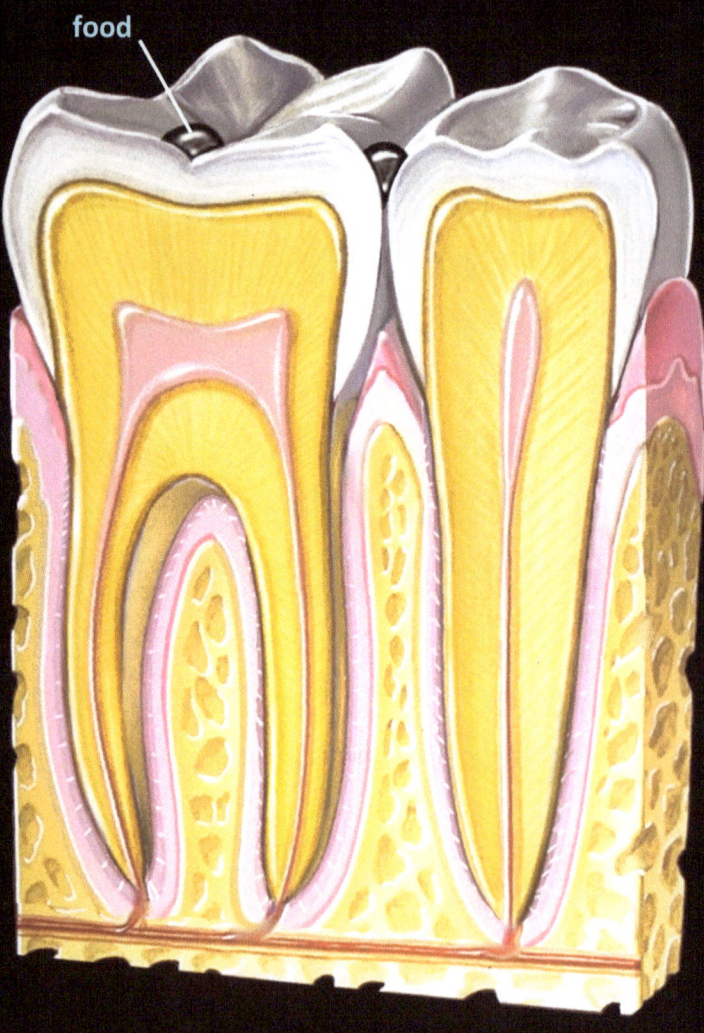

food

Food can become trapped in the crevices of teeth and in between teeth. Bacteria can quickly begin growing in those areas.

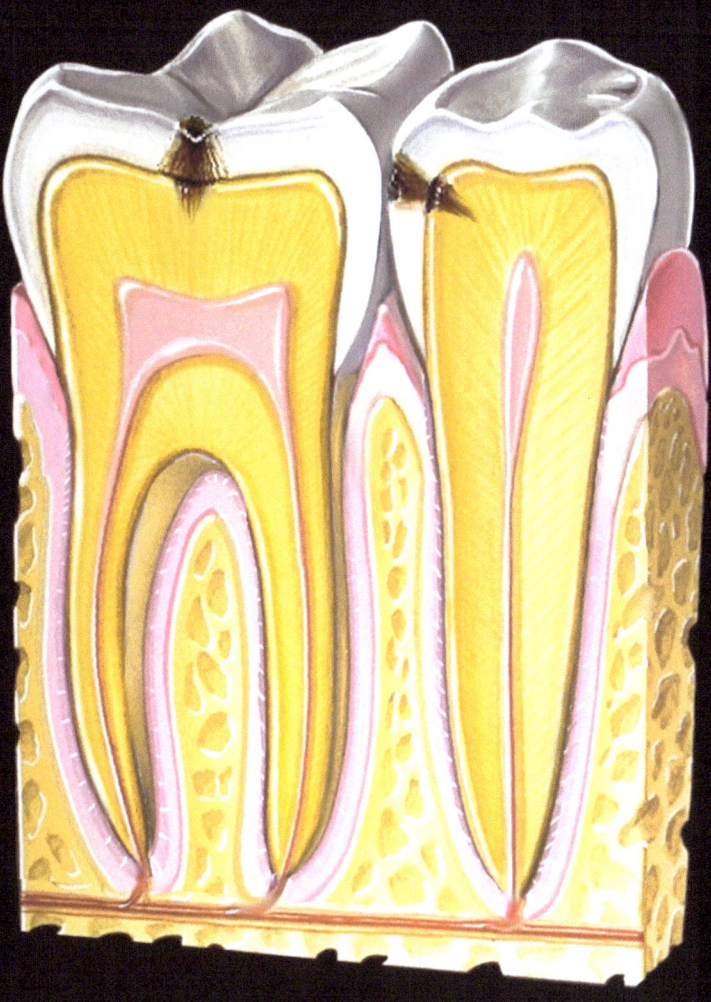

Tooth decay (known as cavities or caries) occurs when acid from bacteria damages the enamel (outer white layer) of a tooth. This decay can progress to the dentin of the tooth (inner yellow layer).

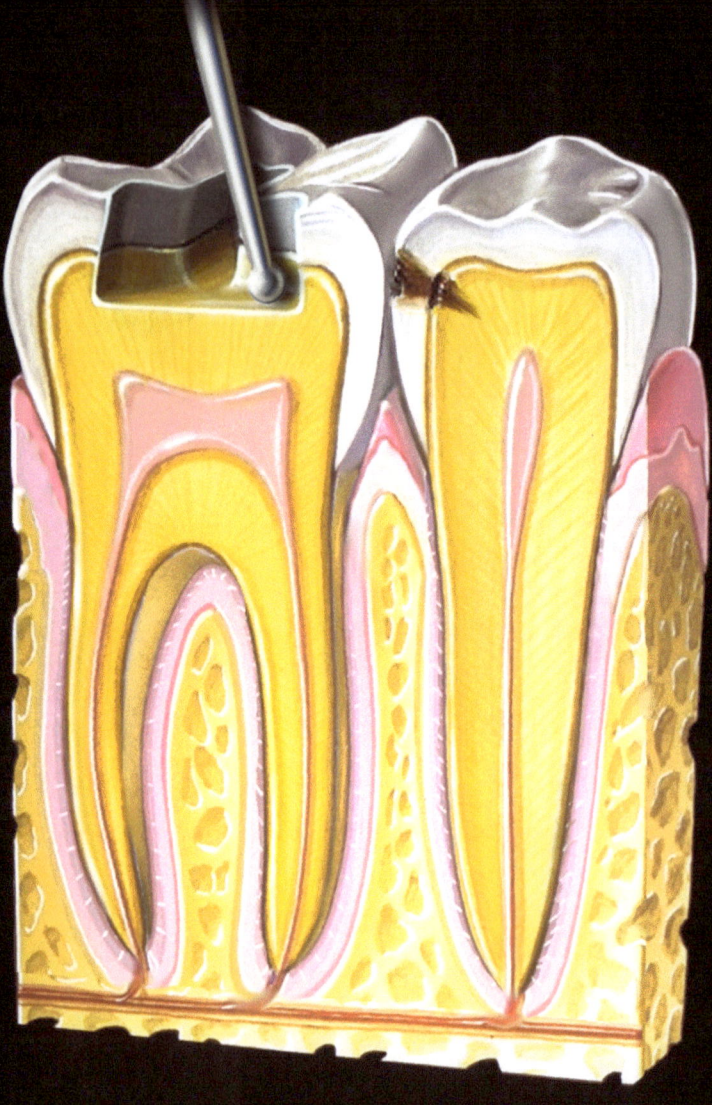

For treatment of caries, the decayed area is removed from both the enamel and dentin.

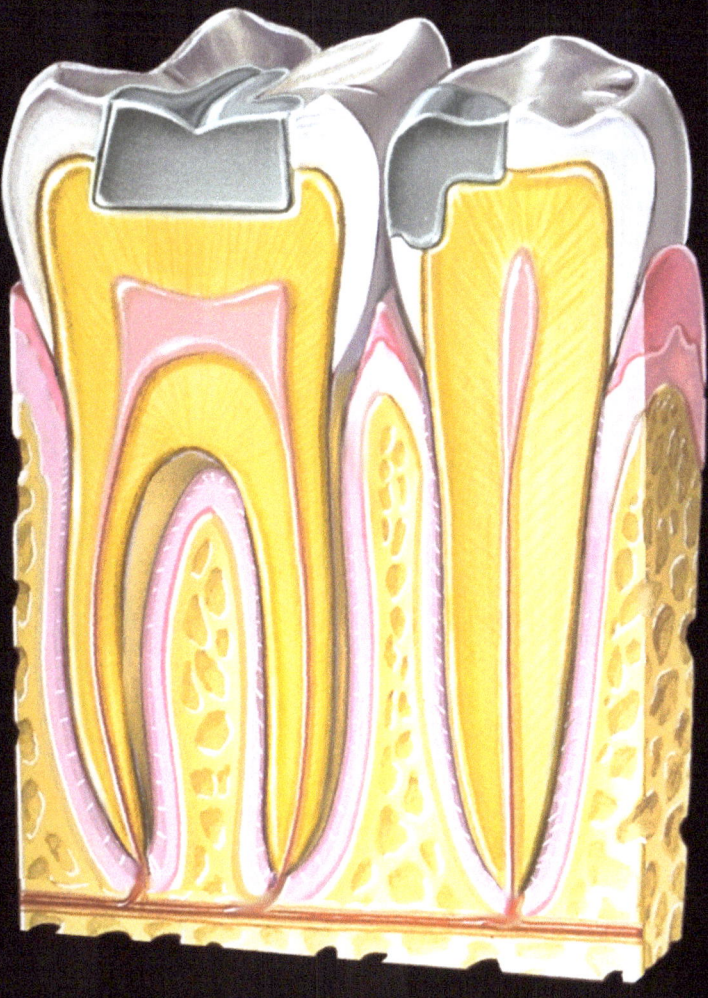

The removed area is replaced with dental amalgam or other filling material.

Root Canal

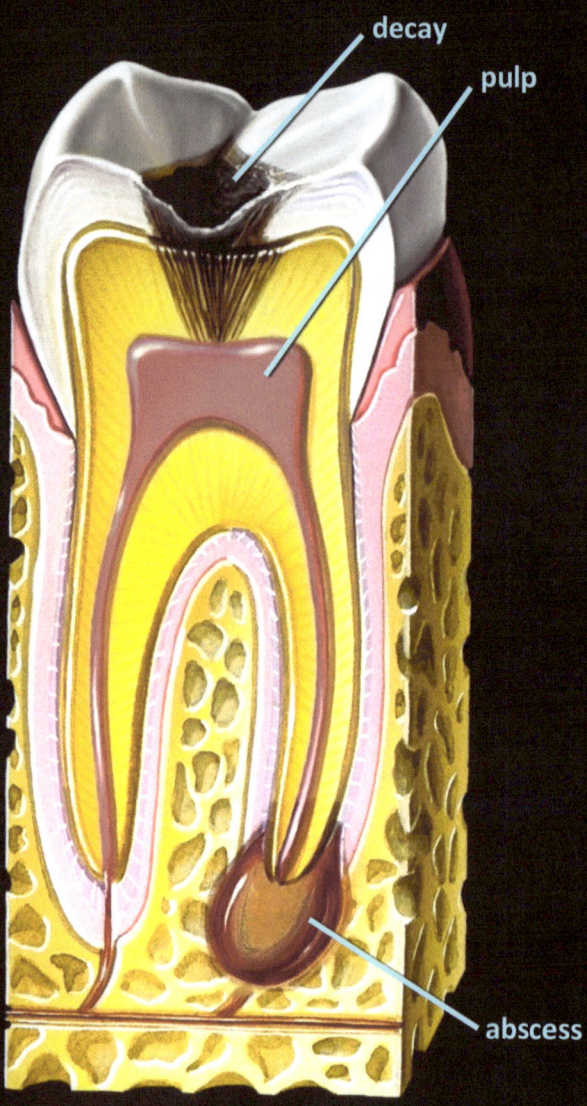

decay

pulp

abscess

Root canal therapy is performed when the living pulp within a tooth becomes infected. An abscess may form at the root tip.

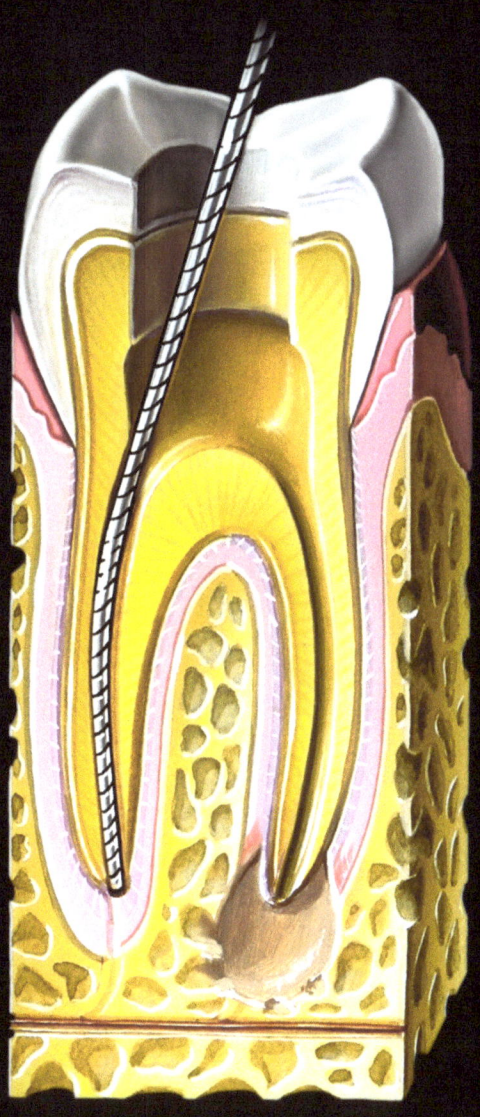

The pulp chamber is opened and cleaned. A special file is used to clean the canals of the tooth roots.

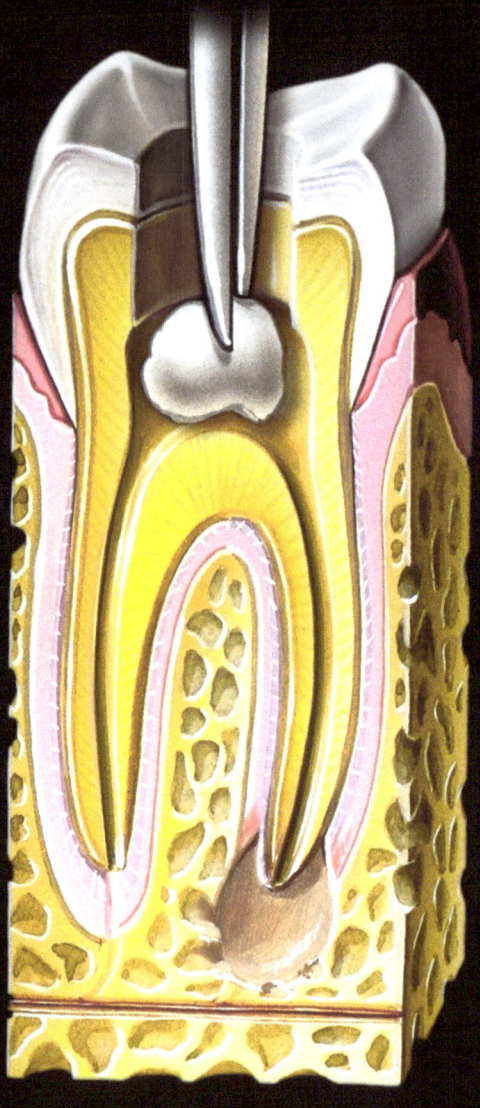

The pulp chamber and root canals are disinfected and then temporarily sealed.

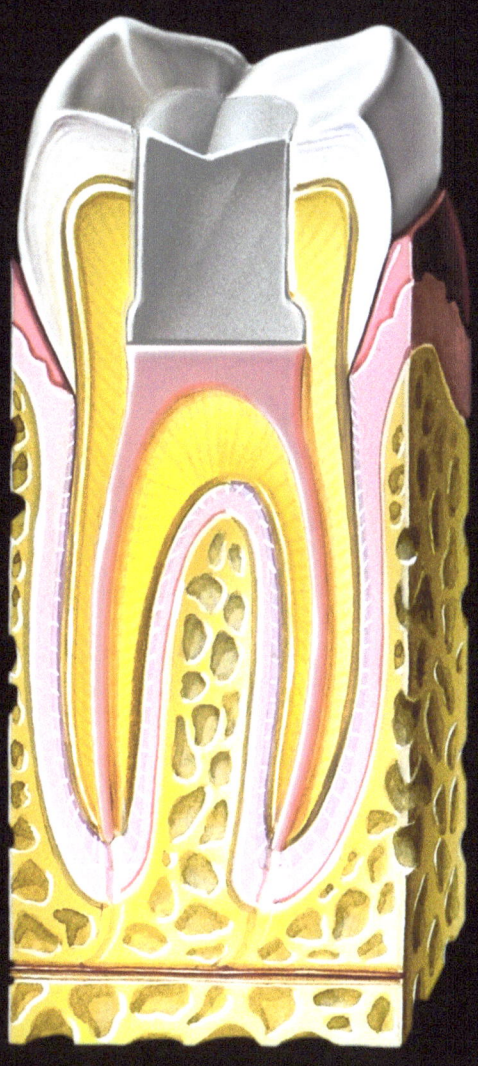

After some time, the canals and pulp chamber are filled
and sealed in a final fashion. A crown may be added
for strength (see Crown).

Periodontal Disease

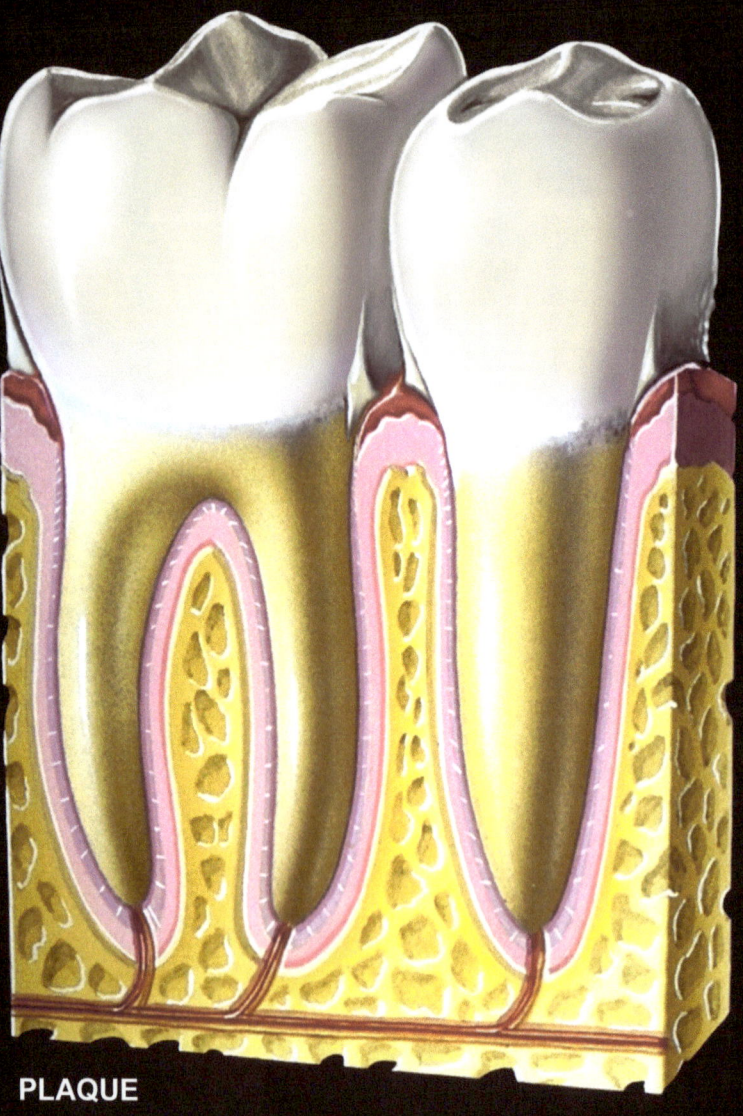

PLAQUE

A sticky white film called plaque can accumulate on teeth and calcify at the gum line to become a hard substance called tartar.

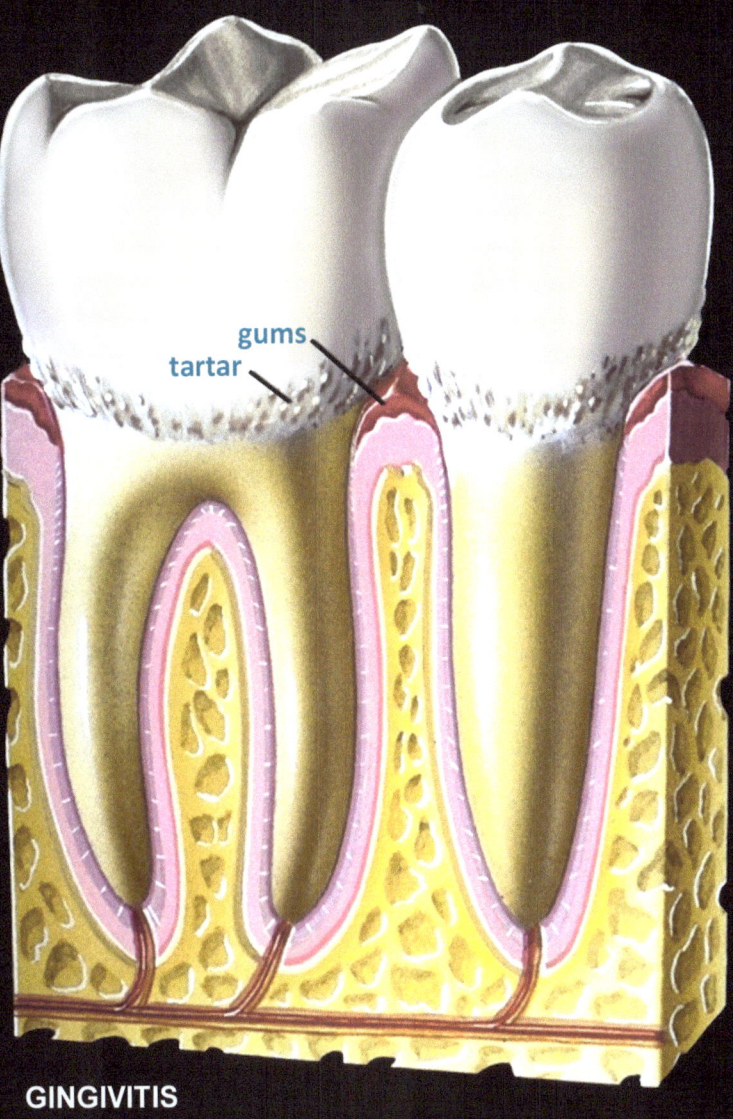

gums
tartar

GINGIVITIS

Build up of tartar can cause inflammation of the gums, called gingivitis.

13

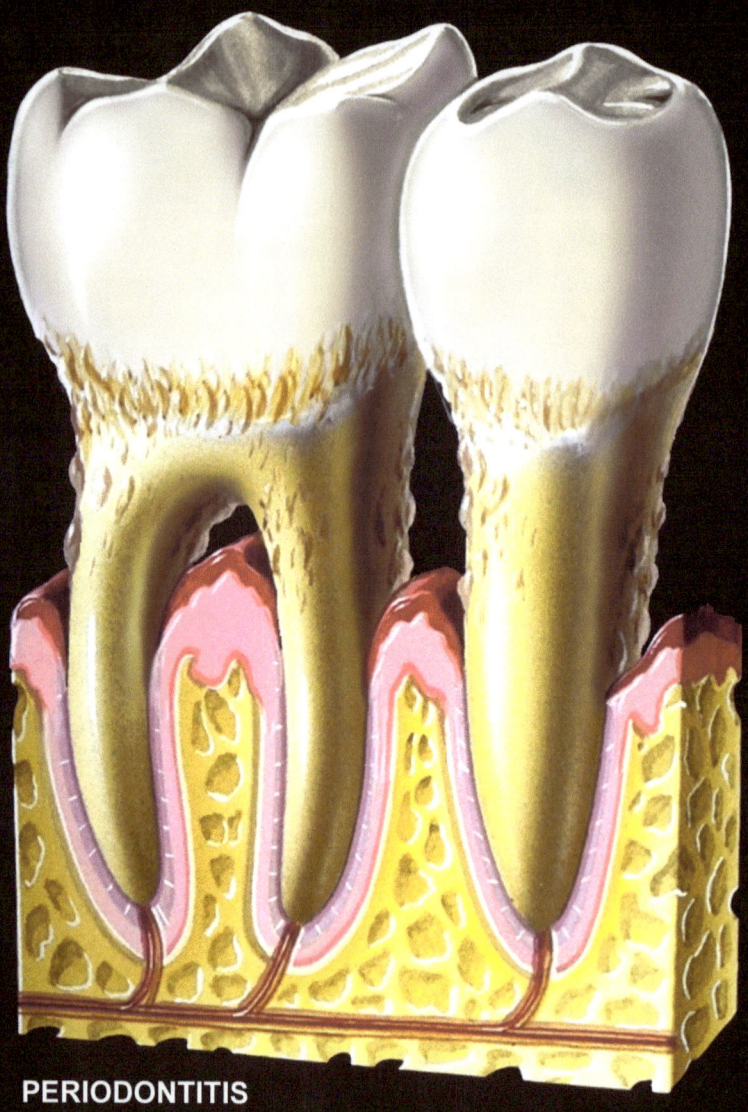

PERIODONTITIS

This can lead to subsequent loss of the bone and ligaments supporting the teeth (periodontitis or Periodontal Disease).

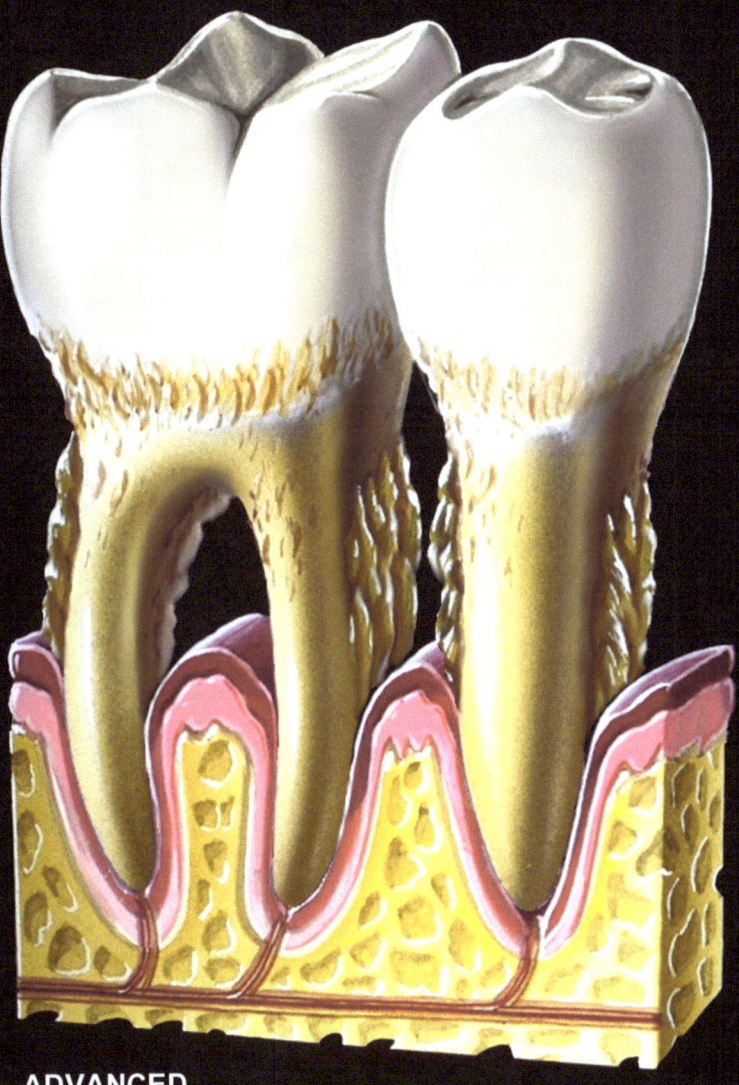

ADVANCED

The teeth can then become loose. Periodontal Disease can lead to eventual loss of the teeth.

15

Pockets & Root Decay

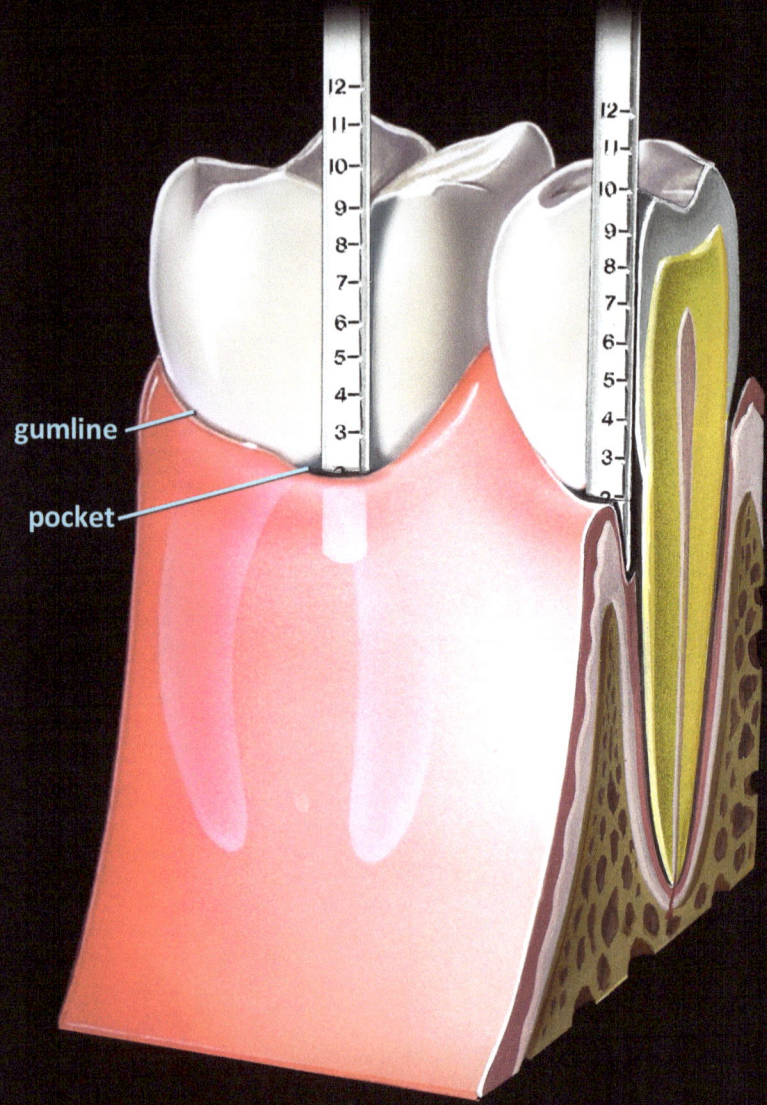

gumline

pocket

At the gumline of each tooth is a small space between the gums and the tooth called the pocket (gingival sulcus). The measured pockets normally have a depth of 1 to 2 mm.

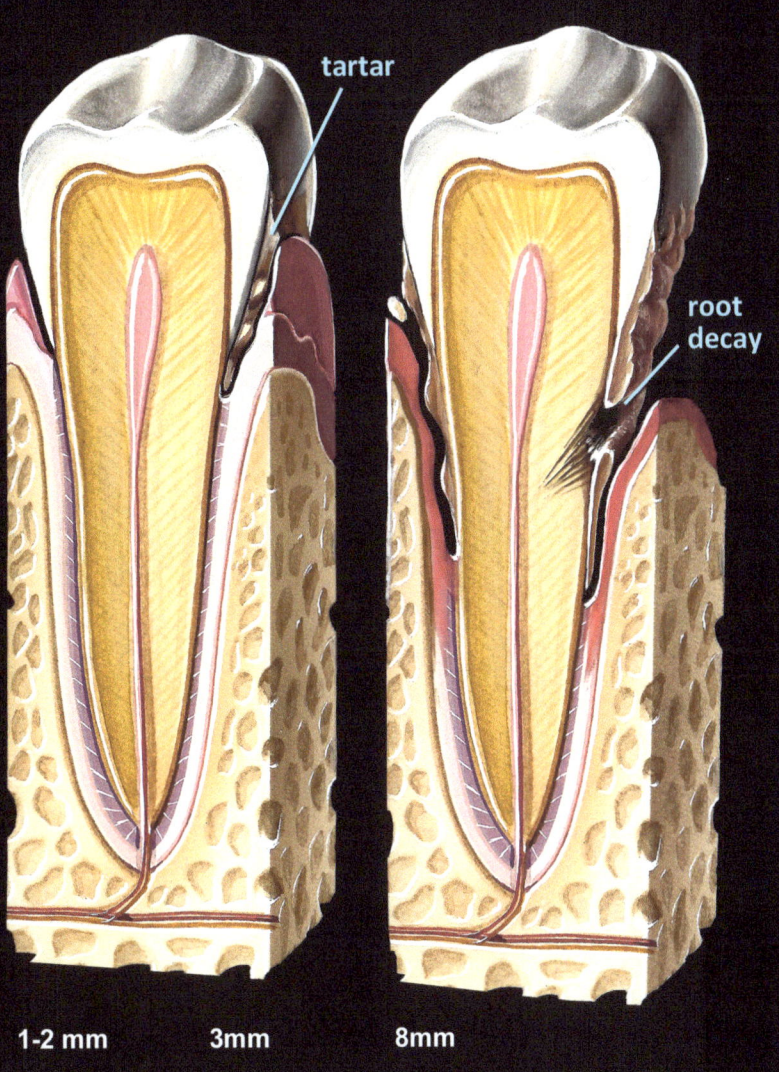

tartar

root decay

1-2 mm   3mm   8mm

Plaque and tartar can build up in the pockets, causing them to deepen. Further build up of plaque and tartar can lead to decay of the root and periodontal disease.

Primary Teeth Caries

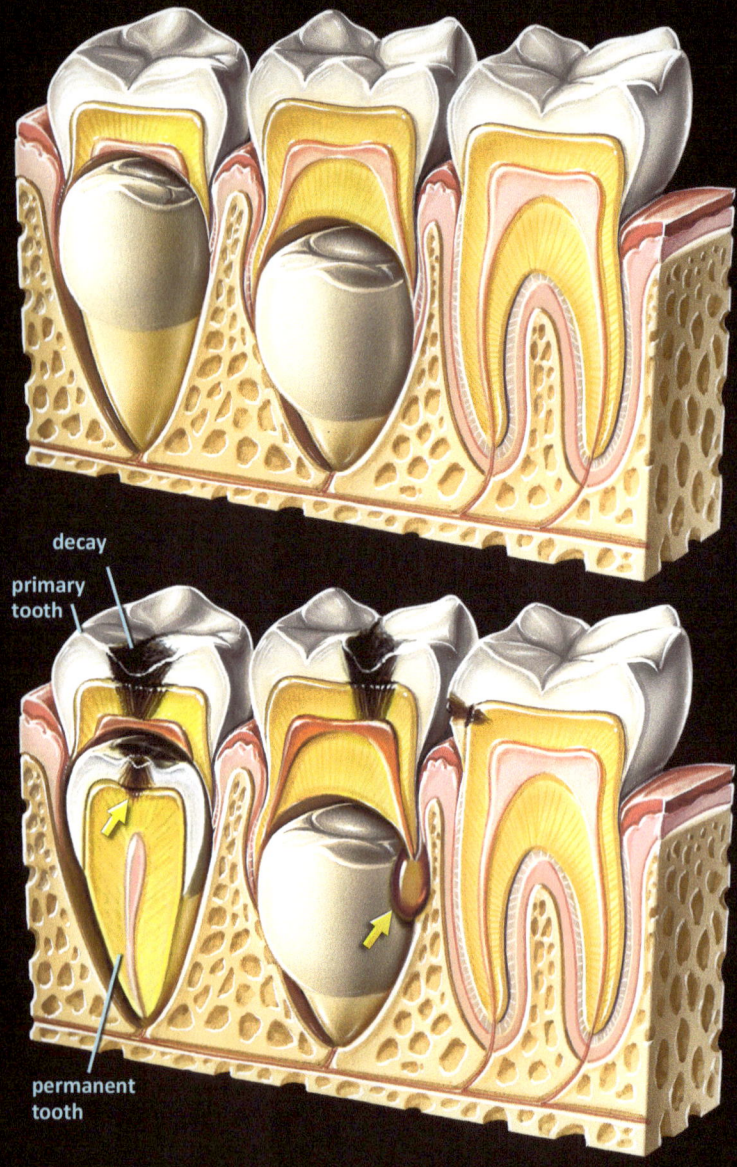

decay

primary tooth

permanent tooth

Dental care and repair of primary teeth is very important to long-term dental health. Primary tooth decay may damage the underlying developing permanent tooth, or cause infection in that area.

18

©1990 Stephen F. Gordon

Gumline Decay

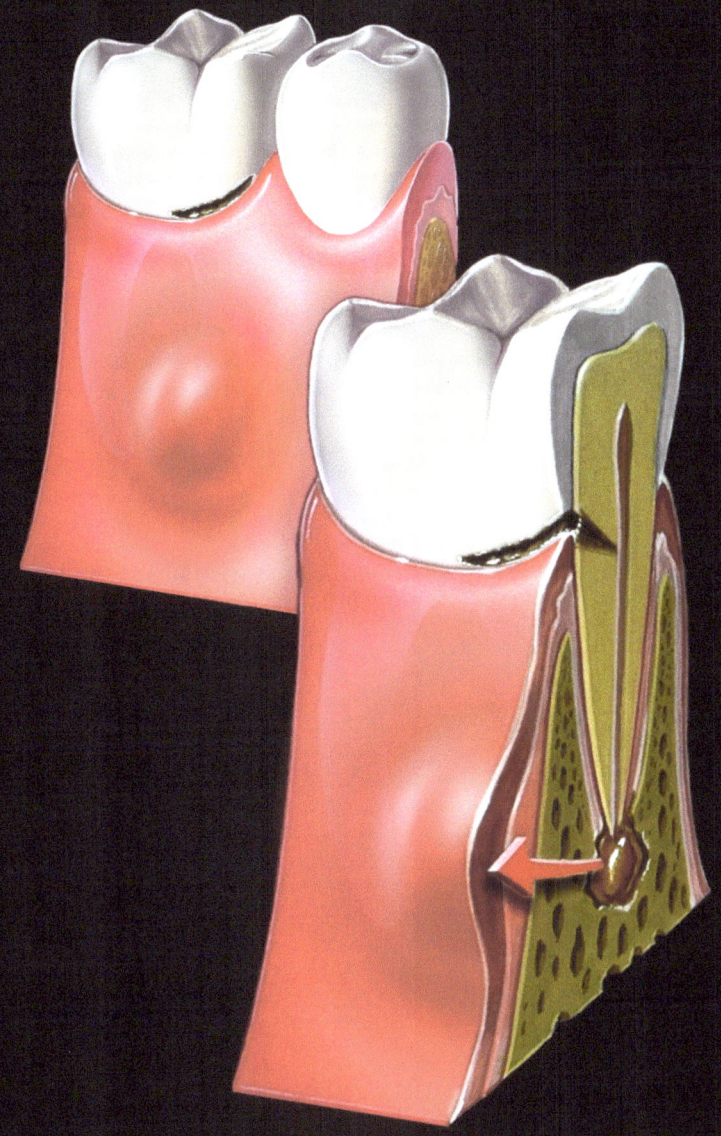

Decay at or below the gumline can cause an infection within the living pulp of the tooth and form an abscess at the root tip. The gums and soft tissue surrounding the tooth will then become swollen and painful.

19

Inlay

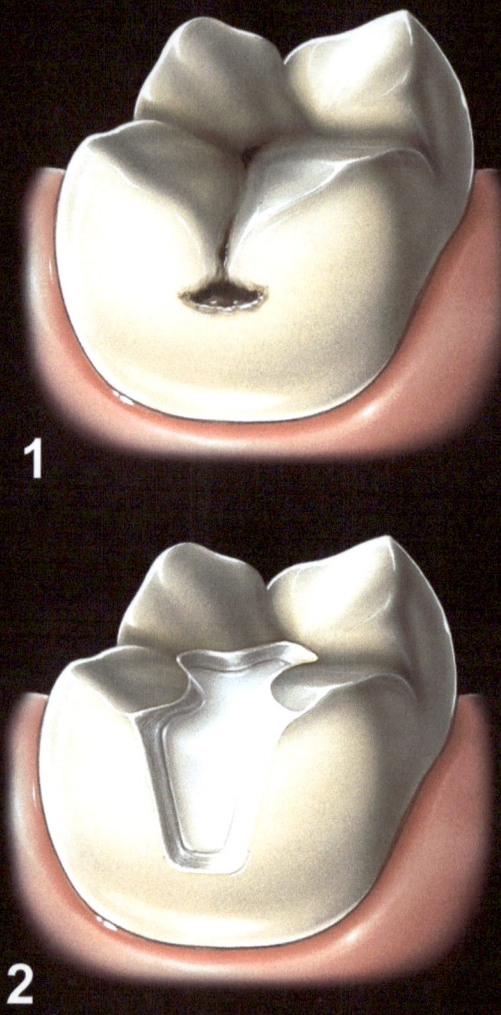

1

2

A dental inlay is used to repair damage to a tooth occurring between the cusps of a tooth (1). The damaged area is prepared by reshaping (2).

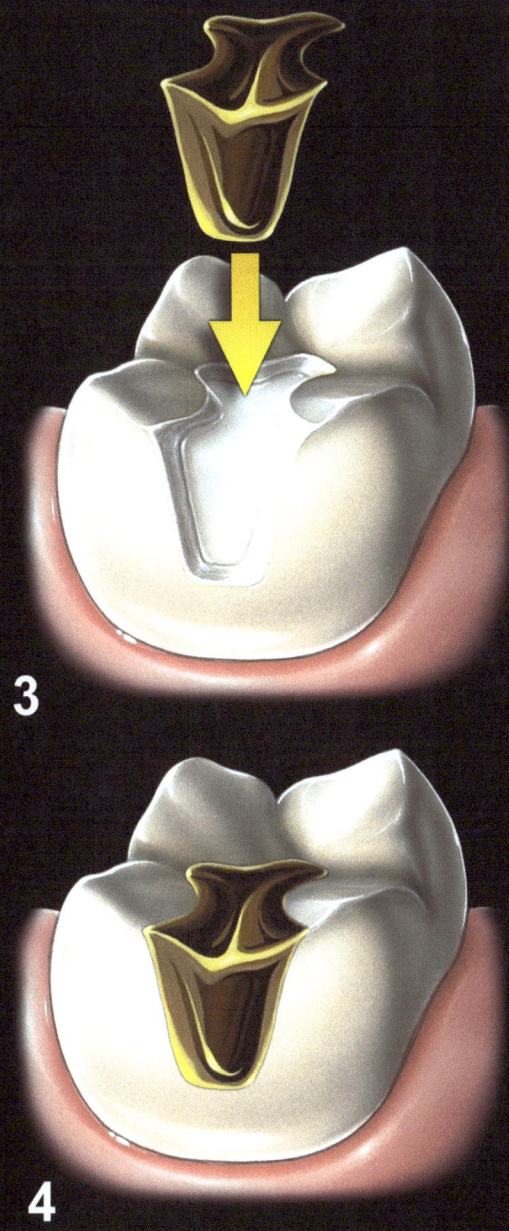

3

4

The custom inlay is affixed to the prepared tooth (3, 4).
Inlays are usually made of composite material, porcelain,
or metal such as gold.

Onlay

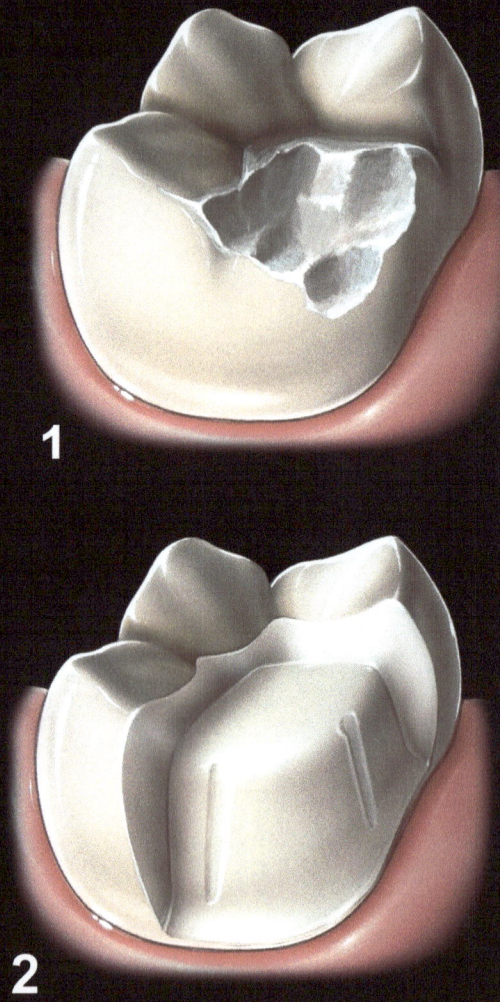

1

2

A dental onlay is used to repair a cracked or broken cusp of a tooth (1). The damaged area is reshaped (2).

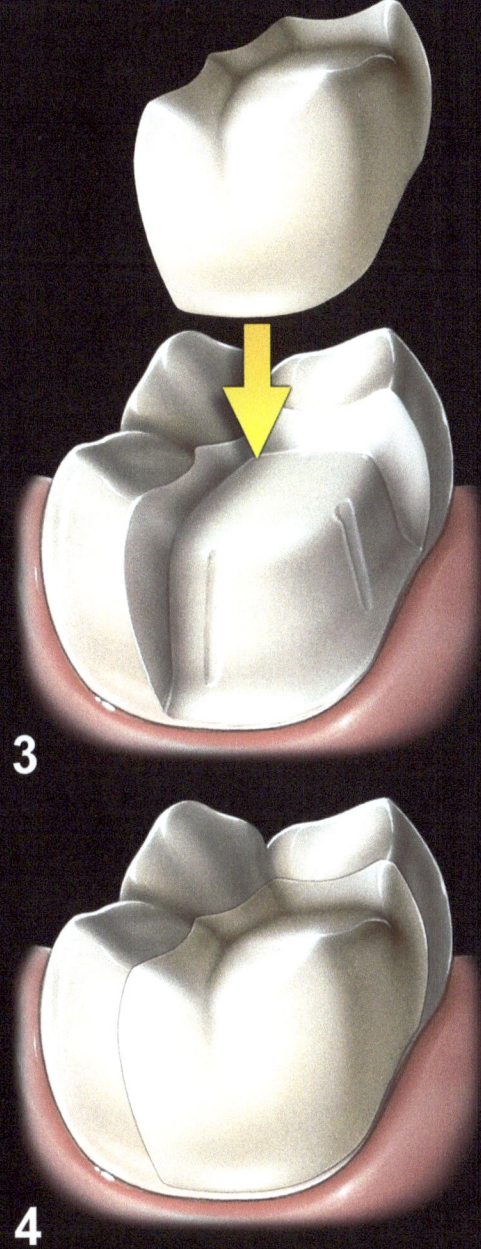

3

4

The custom onlay is affixed to the prepared tooth (3, 4).
Onlays are usually made of composite material or
porcelain.

23

Crown

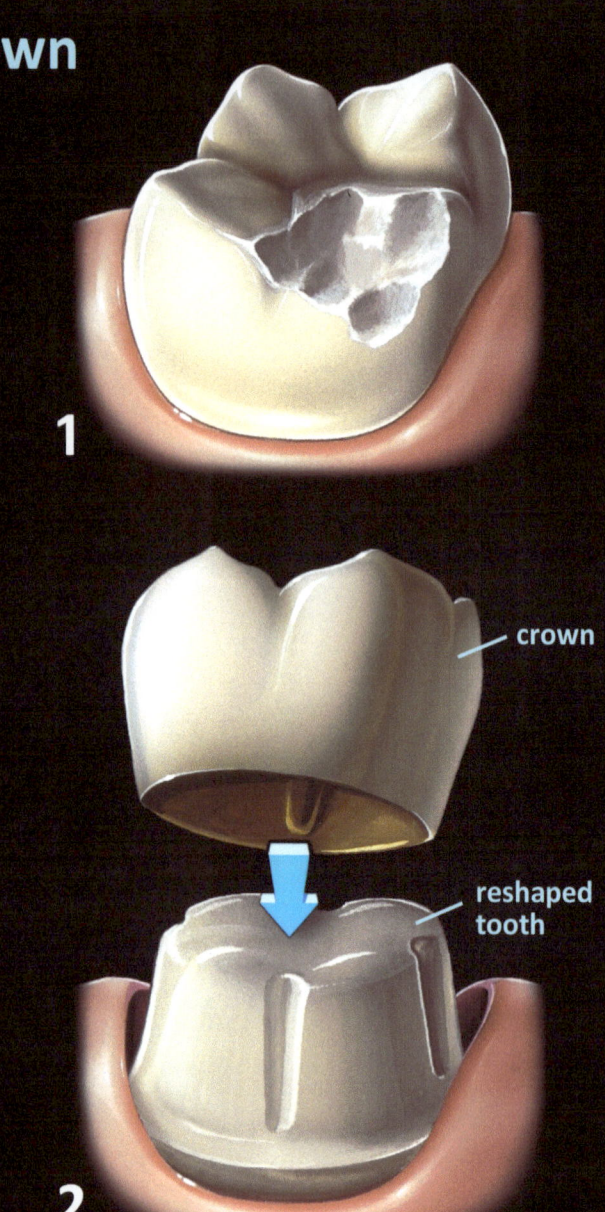

1

crown

reshaped
tooth

2

A crown is a tooth-shaped restoration placed over an existing weak, broken, or unattractive tooth **(1)**. The original tooth is reshaped **(2)** and usually covered by a temporary crown while the final crown is prepared.

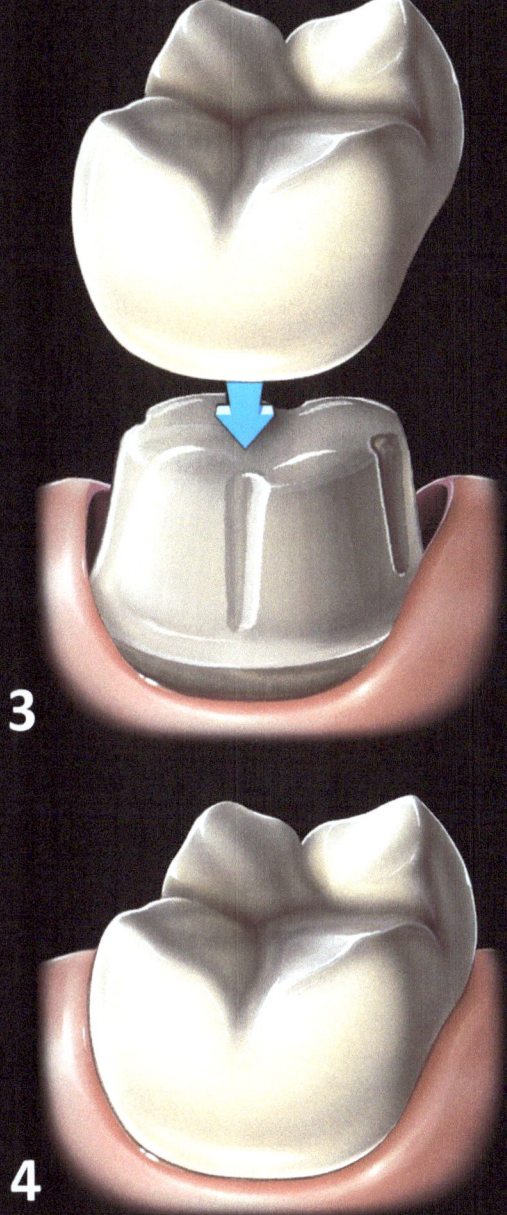

3

4

The temporary crown is removed and the final crown is cemented onto the reshaped tooth (3,4). A crown may also be used to protect and strengthen a tooth which has undergone root canal therapy.

25

Bridge

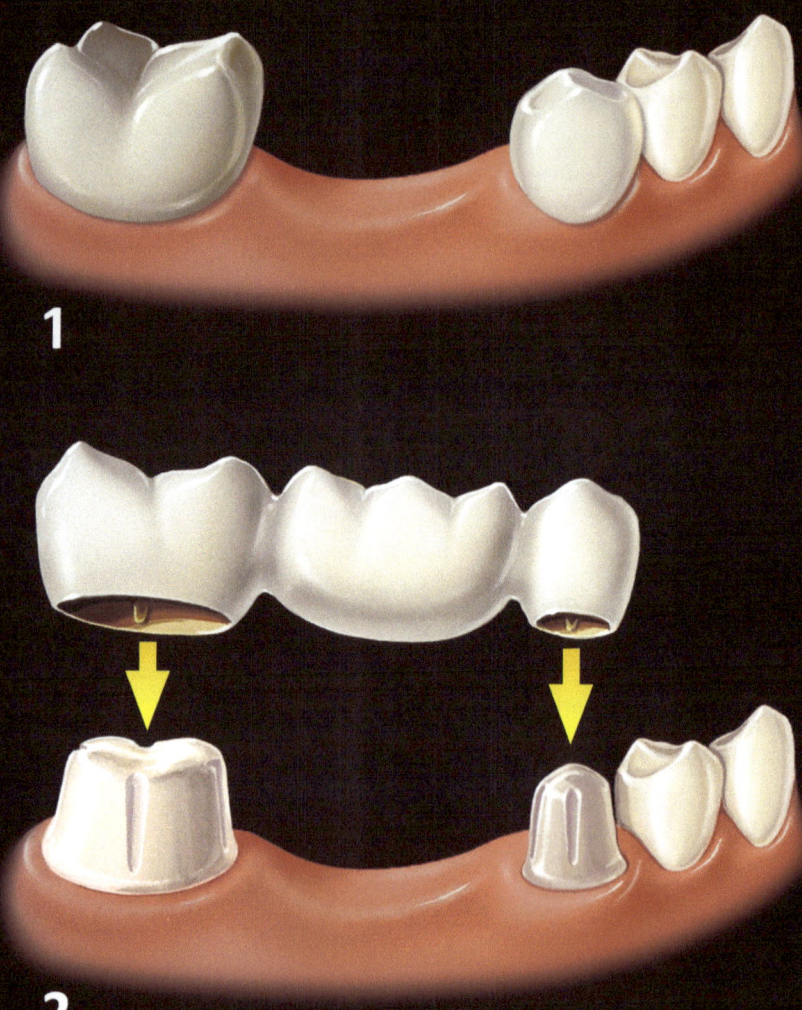

1

2

A fixed bridge is a dental restoration designed to span the space of a missing tooth (**1**). The teeth on each side of the space are reshaped, and the bridge is affixed onto them.

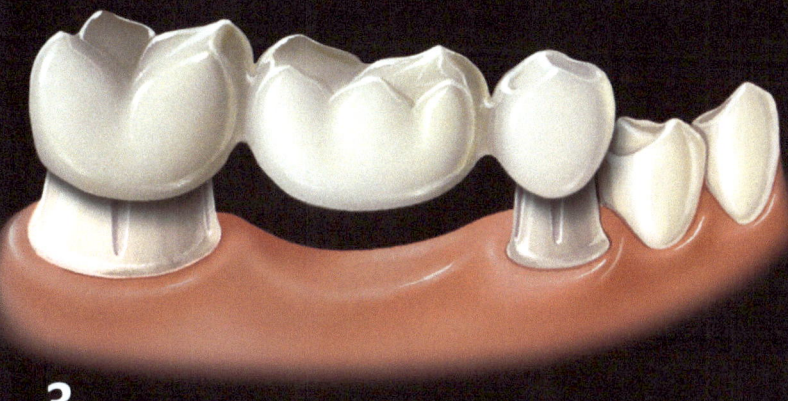

3

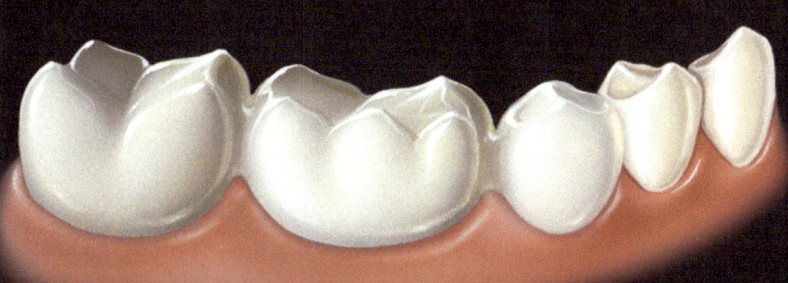

4

The bridge is shown moving into position on the reshaped teeth (3,4). The bridge is cemented onto the reshaped teeth to become fixed.

Maryland Bridge

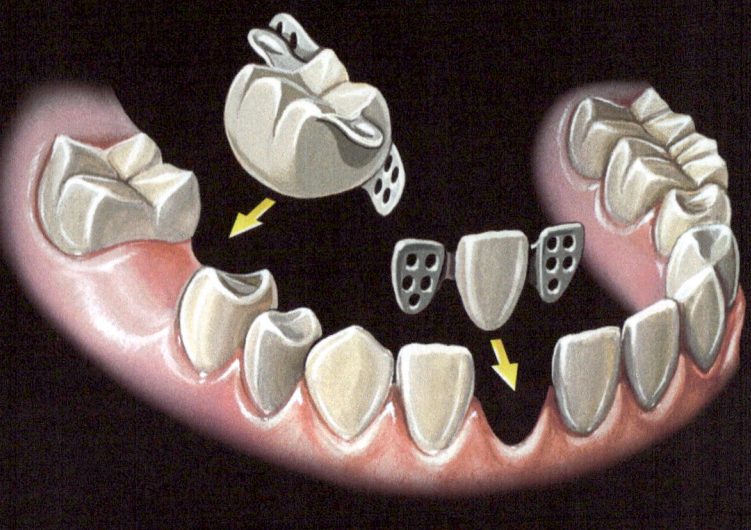

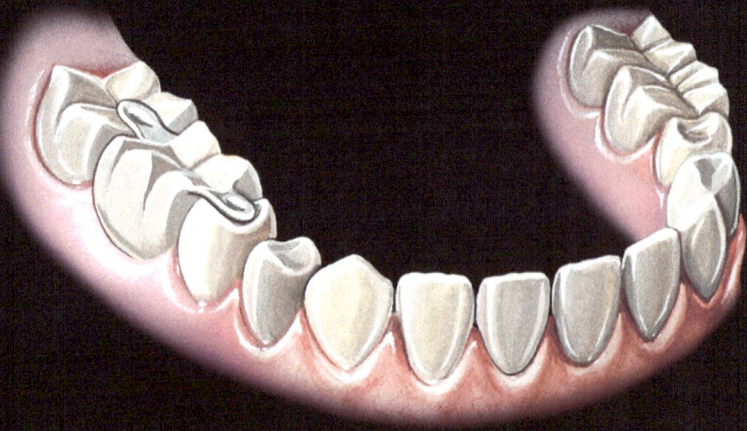

A Maryland Bridge is a custom-designed restoration for replacing a missing tooth. It generally consists of an artificial tooth with metal wings. The wings adhere to the back or top of adjoining teeth to hide them.

Removable Partial Denture

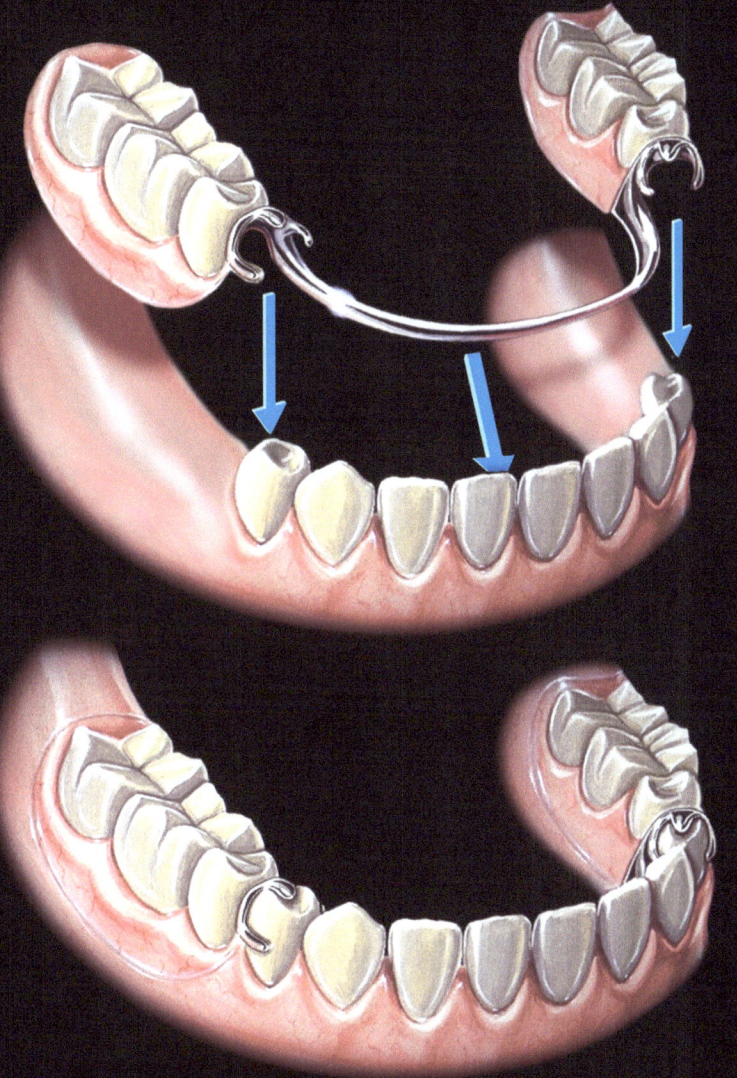

A removable partial denture is a custom-designed restoration used to replace groups of missing teeth. It may be held in place by clasps, and the supporting metal is hidden behind teeth when possible.

29

Implants

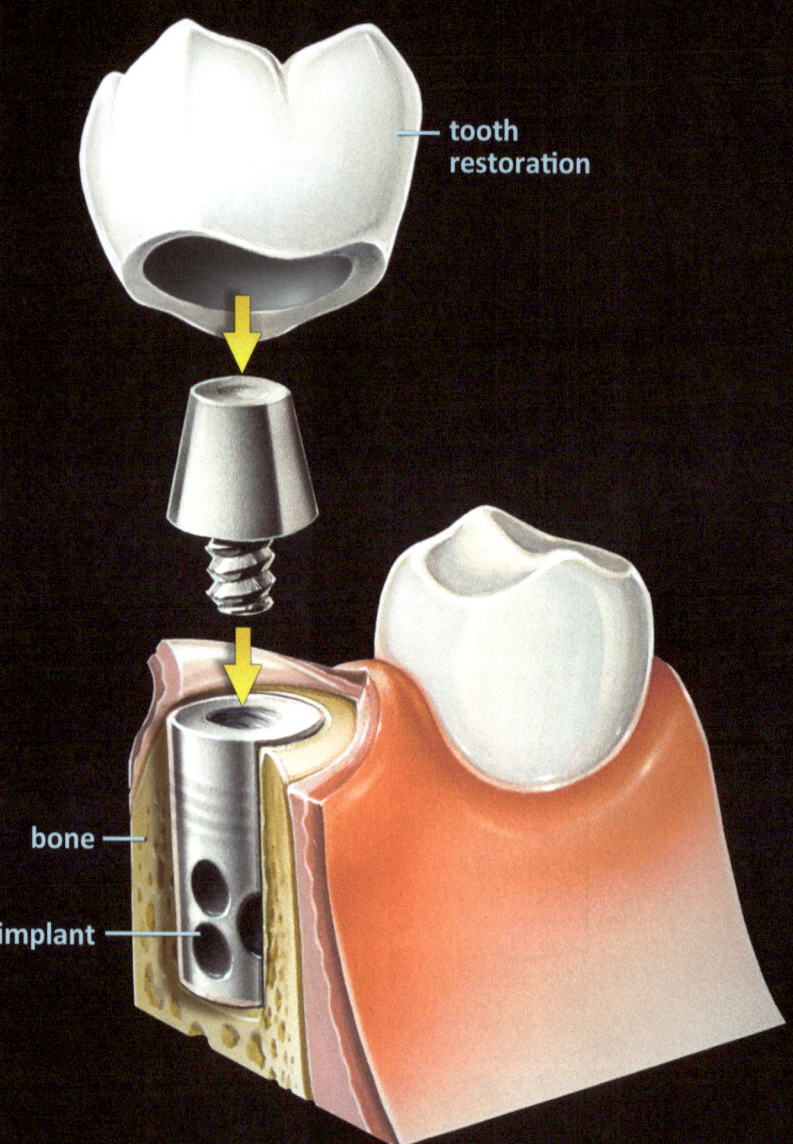

tooth restoration

bone

implant

A dental implant is an artificial supportive root placed within the jaw bone. Implants are used in cases of a missing tooth or teeth.

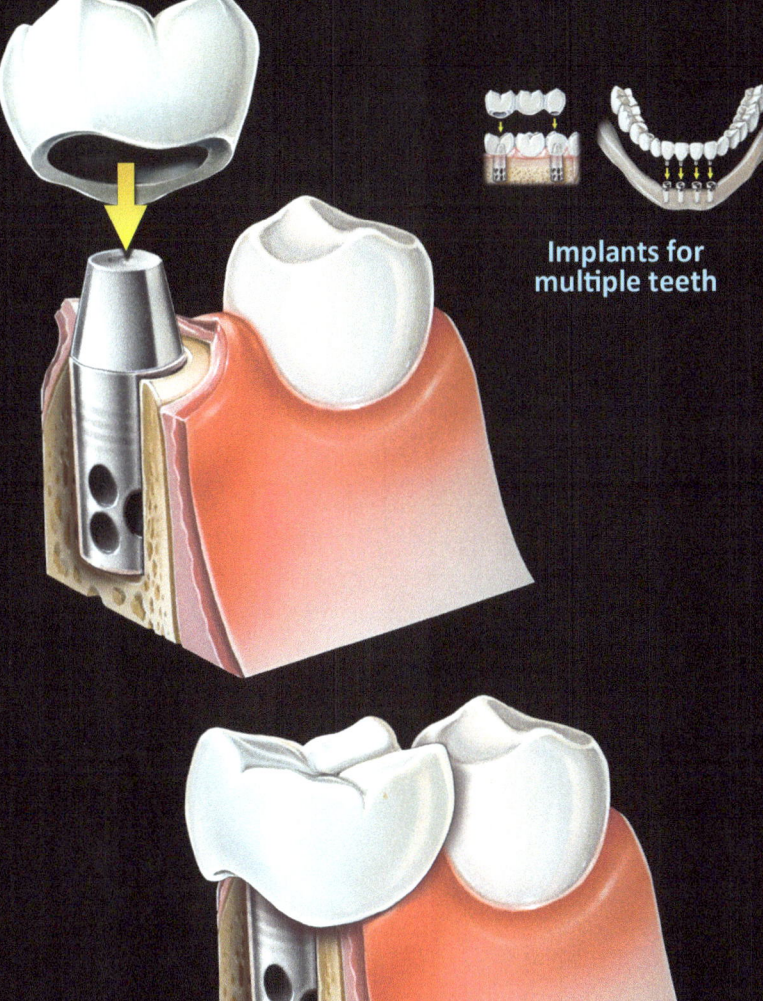

Implants for multiple teeth

The implant fuses with the bone over time (called osseointegration). A tooth restoration is then affixed onto the implant.

31

Pins, Posts & Cores

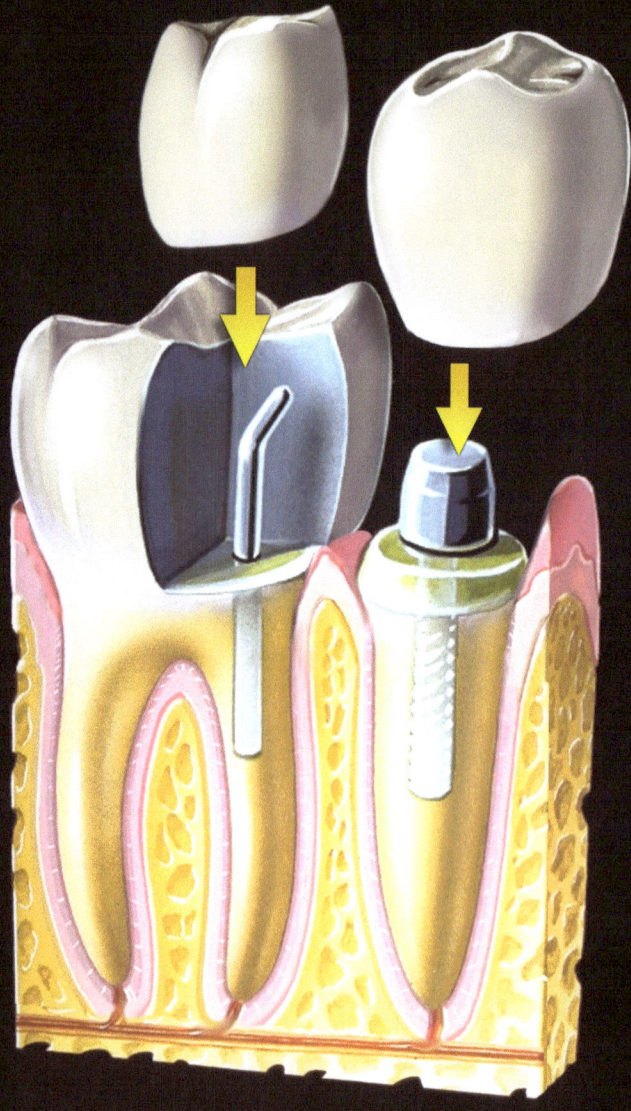

In cases where a large portion of a tooth has become damaged or broken, a partial tooth restoration may be affixed more securely when combined with a metal pin or post preplaced within the core of the original tooth.

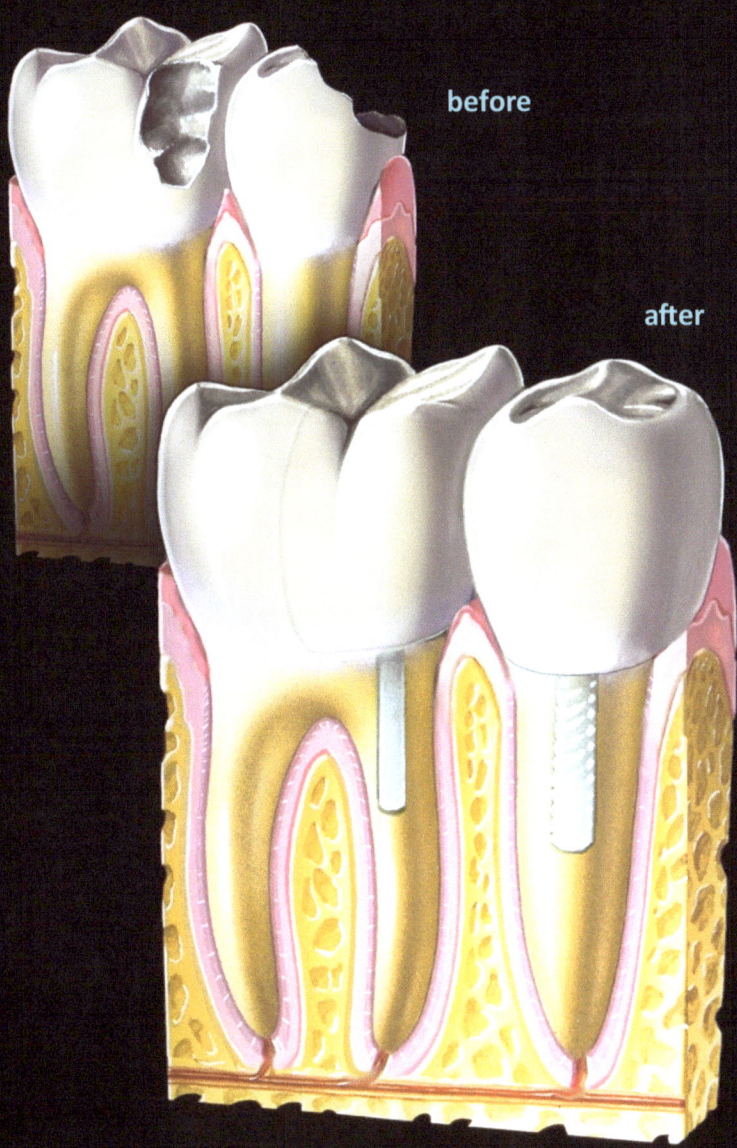

before

after

Shown above are the damaged teeth before, and the restored teeth after, using pins and posts (ghost view) to firmly secure the restorations.

Bonding

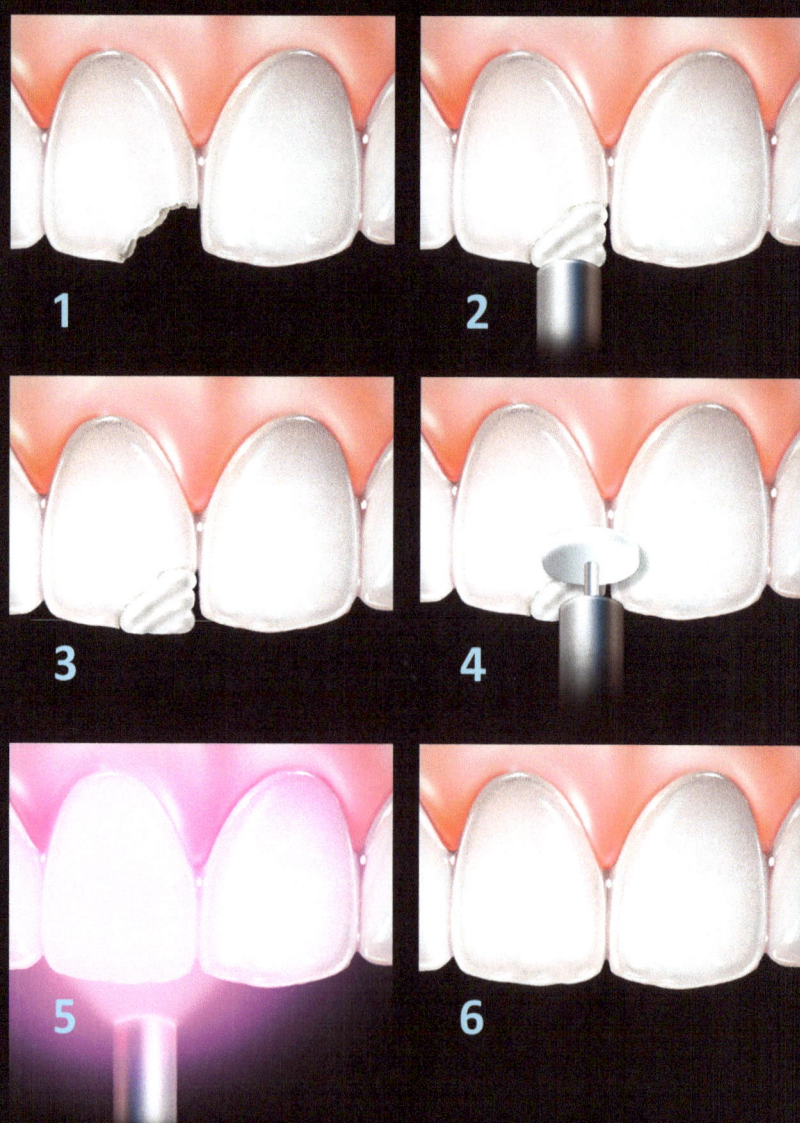

Bonding may be used to restore chipped teeth (1) or fill spaces between teeth. A strong composite material is added to the prepared tooth (2,3), where it is shaped (4), and cured with a special light (5). The chip is repaired (6).

Veneers

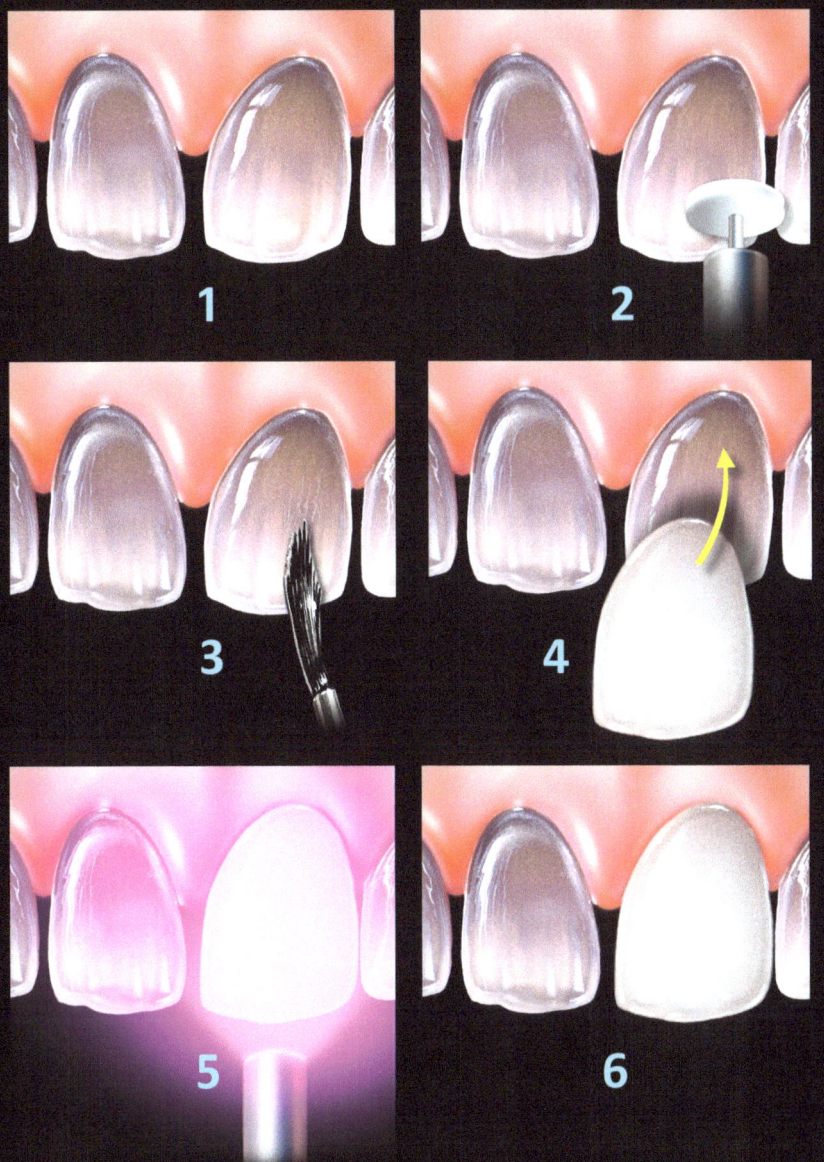

A tooth-shaped covering, or veneer, is affixed onto the front surface of a discolored or worn tooth (1). The tooth surface is prepared (2) and etched (3). Special light cures an adhesive (4,5), affixing the veneer to the tooth (6).

Sealants

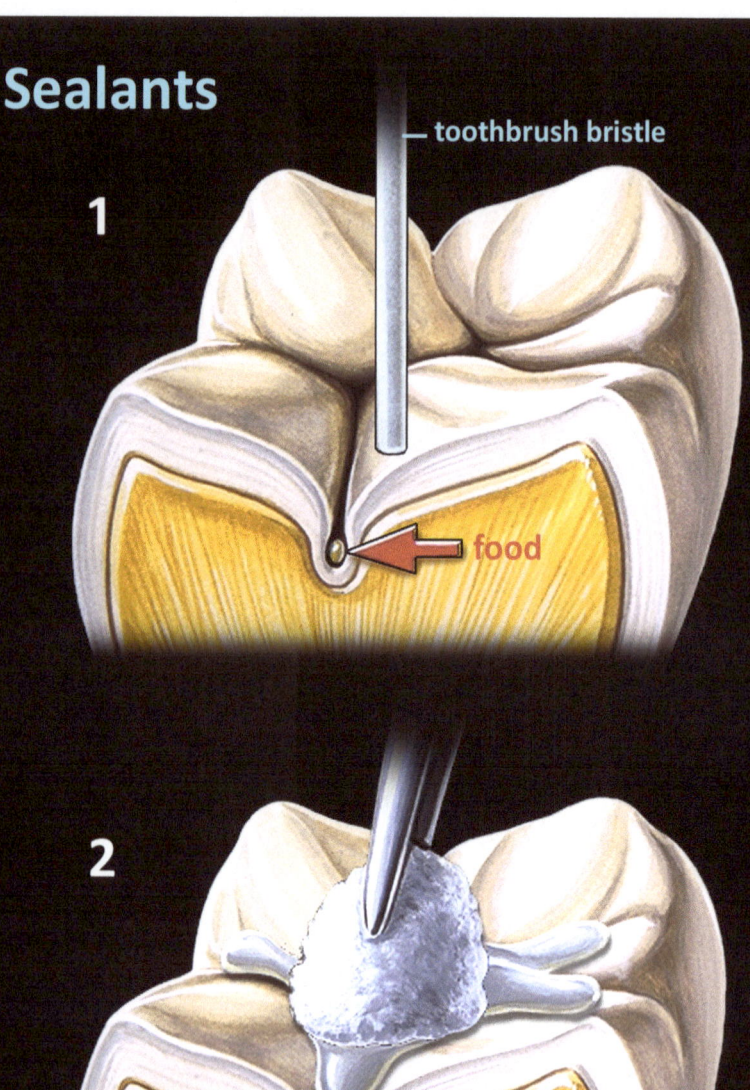

1

— toothbrush bristle

food

2

Sealants are a protective material used to fill areas of the teeth which are prone to tooth decay, such as crevices of molars where food typically becomes trapped (1). The sealant material is applied to the teeth in liquid form (2).

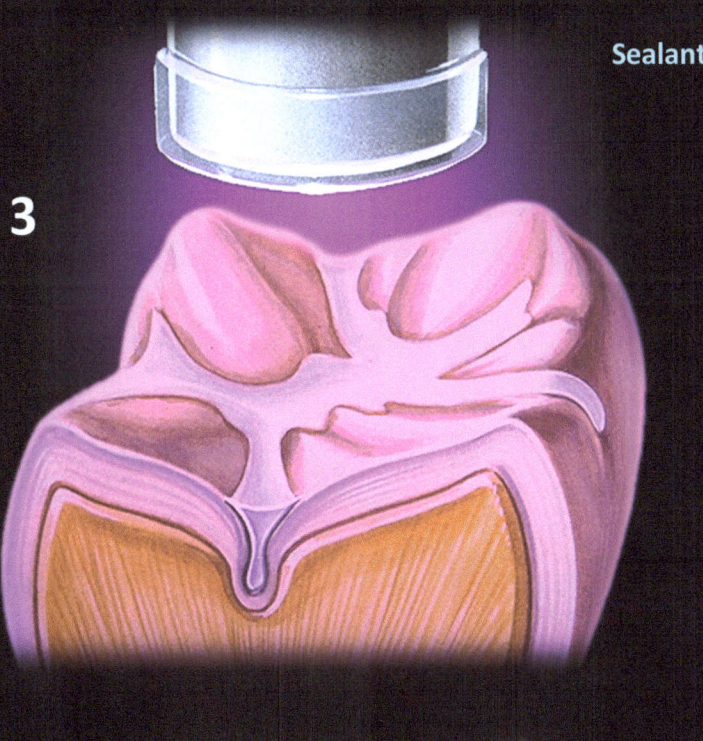

3

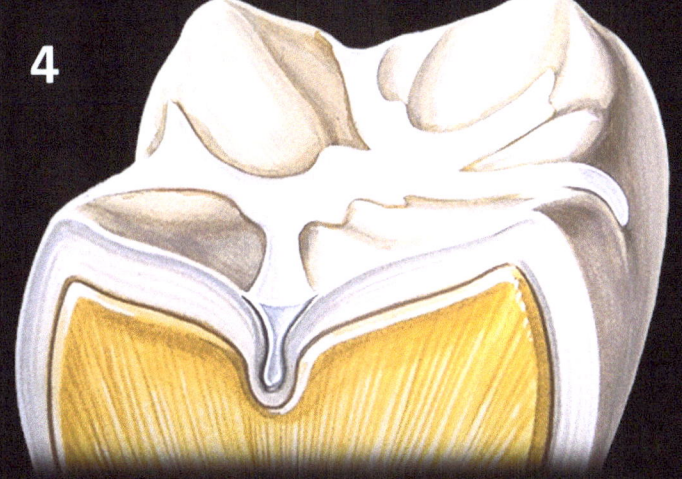

4

The sealant material is then hardened using a special light **(3)**. Food is now effectively blocked from entering the tooth crevices **(4)**.

Impaction

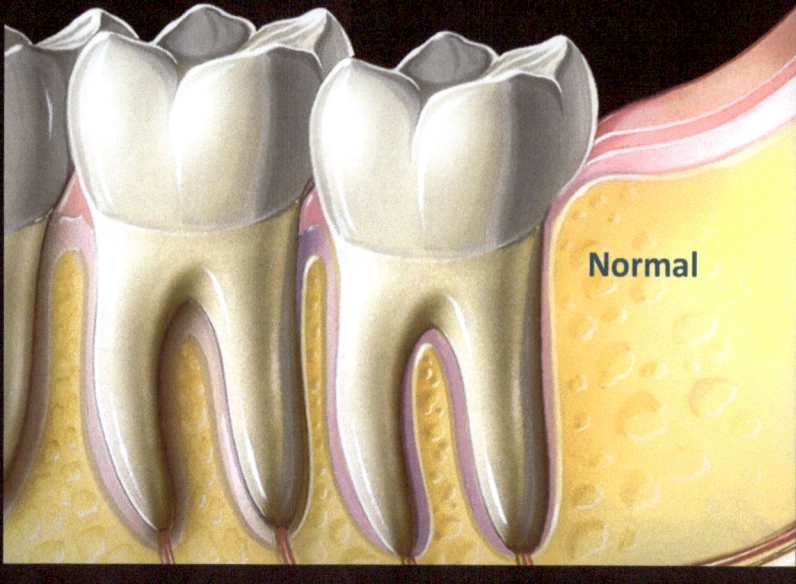

Normal

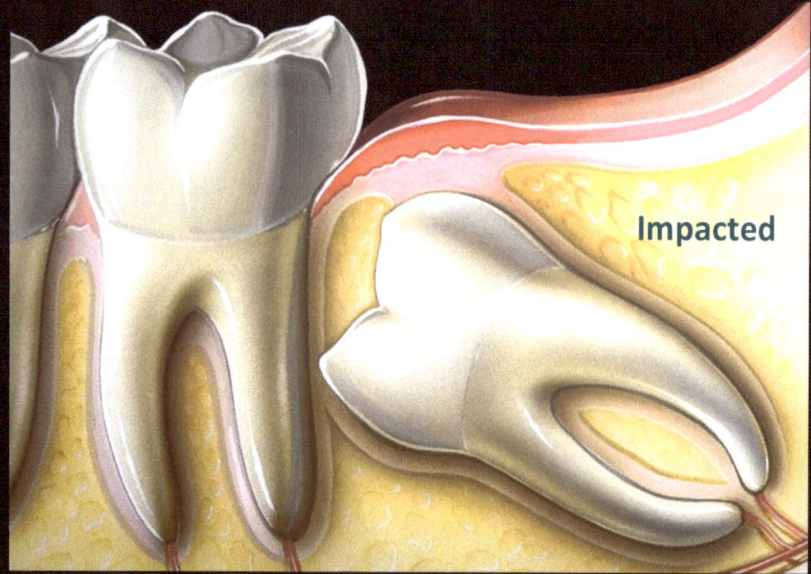

Impacted

A tooth may become blocked from emerging to a normal position by an adjacent tooth, surrounding bone, or soft tissue. The example shown is a wisdom tooth (3rd molar) that is impacted, requiring surgical removal.

Diastemata

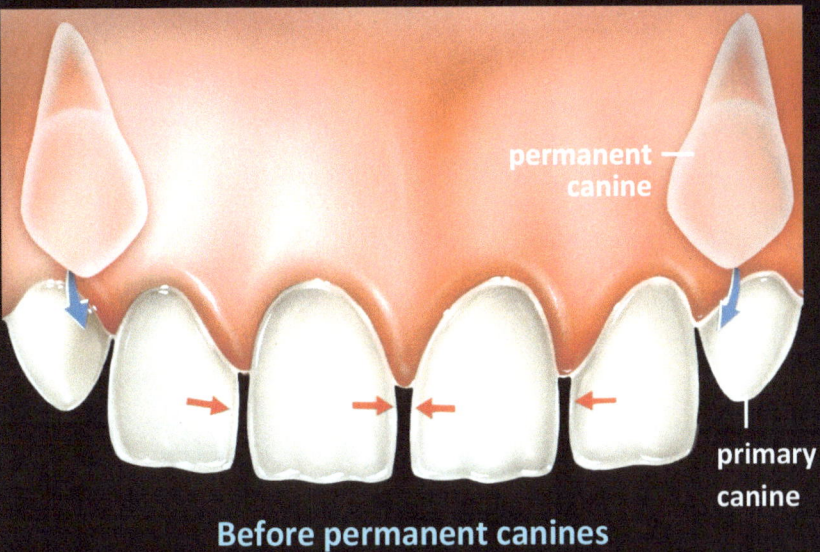

permanent canine

primary canine

Before permanent canines

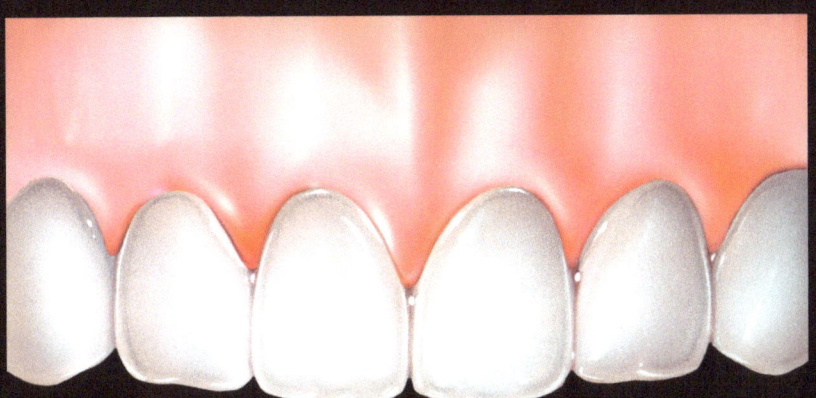

After permanent canines

Before the permanent canines appear, children may have spaces (diastemas-red arrows) between their permanent incisors. This usually remedies itself once the larger permanent canines erupt, pushing the incisors together.

TMJ (temporomandibular joint)

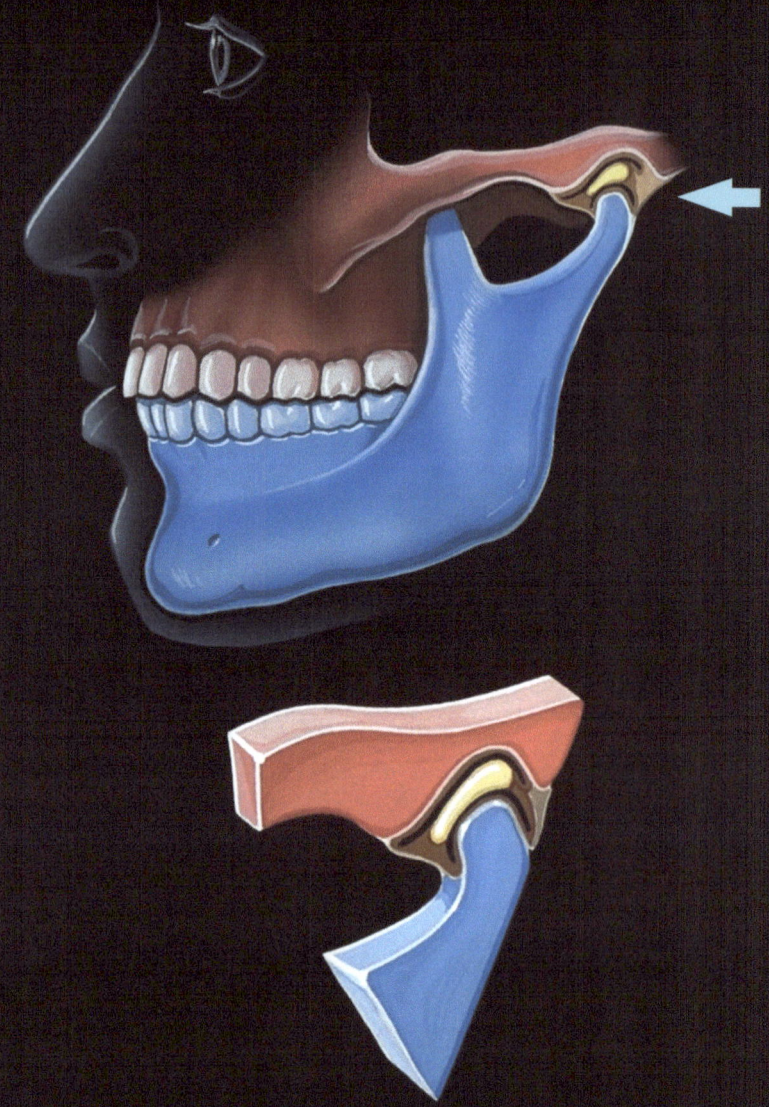

TMJ refers to the Temporomandibular Joint located between the movable lower jaw (lower mandible - blue) and fixed upper jaw (upper mandible - red) of the skull.

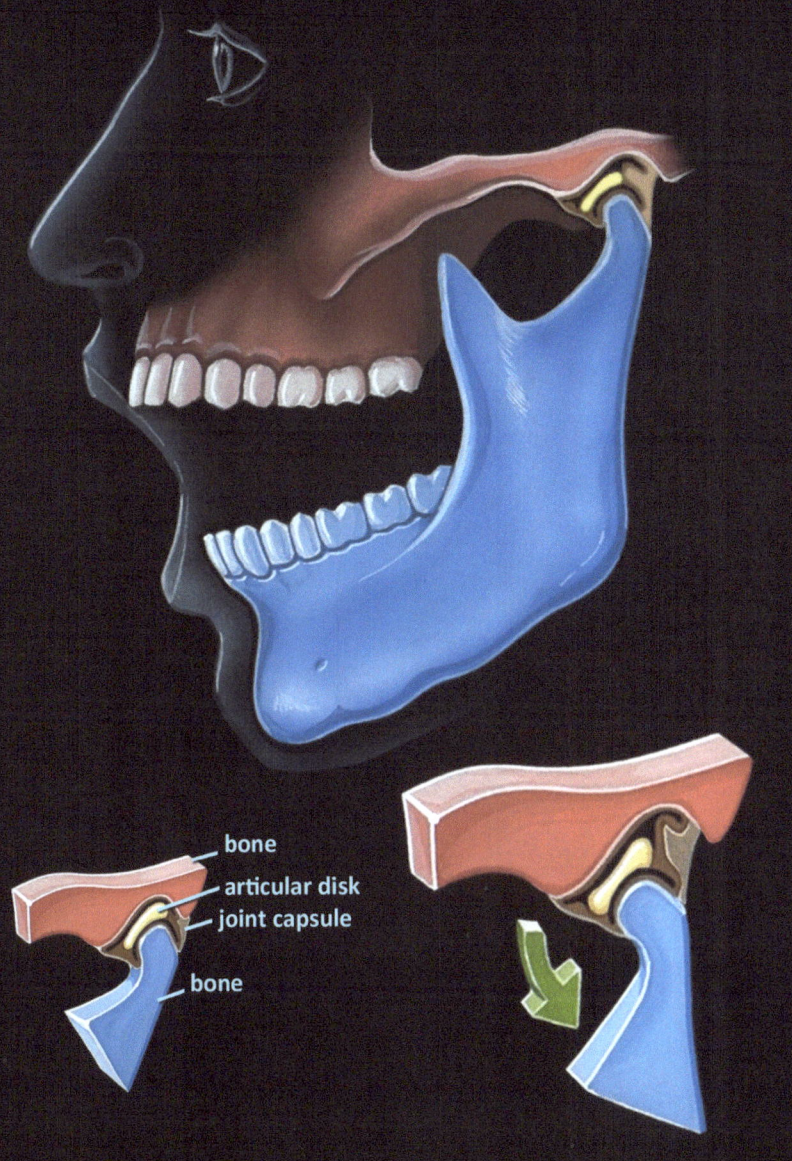

bone
articular disk
joint capsule
bone

The joint primarily consists of bone, fibrous joint capsule, and the articular disk. There are variety of disorders which can affect this very important joint.

41

Postive Effects - New Denture

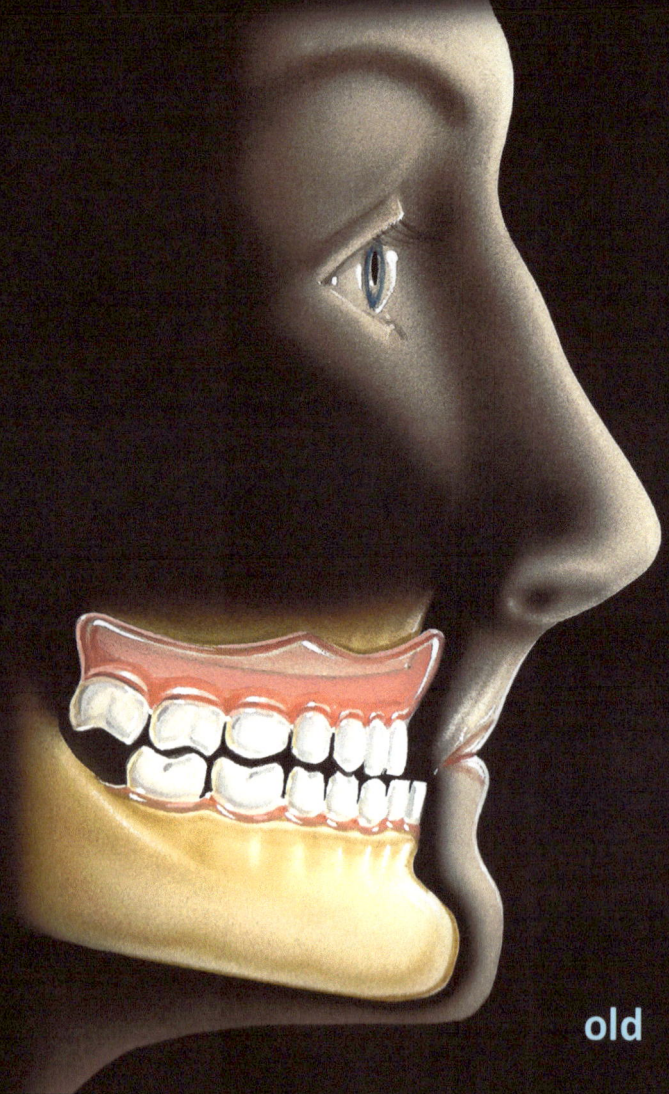

old

Changes in ones gums and jaw bones over time can cause a denture to not fit properly and become loose.

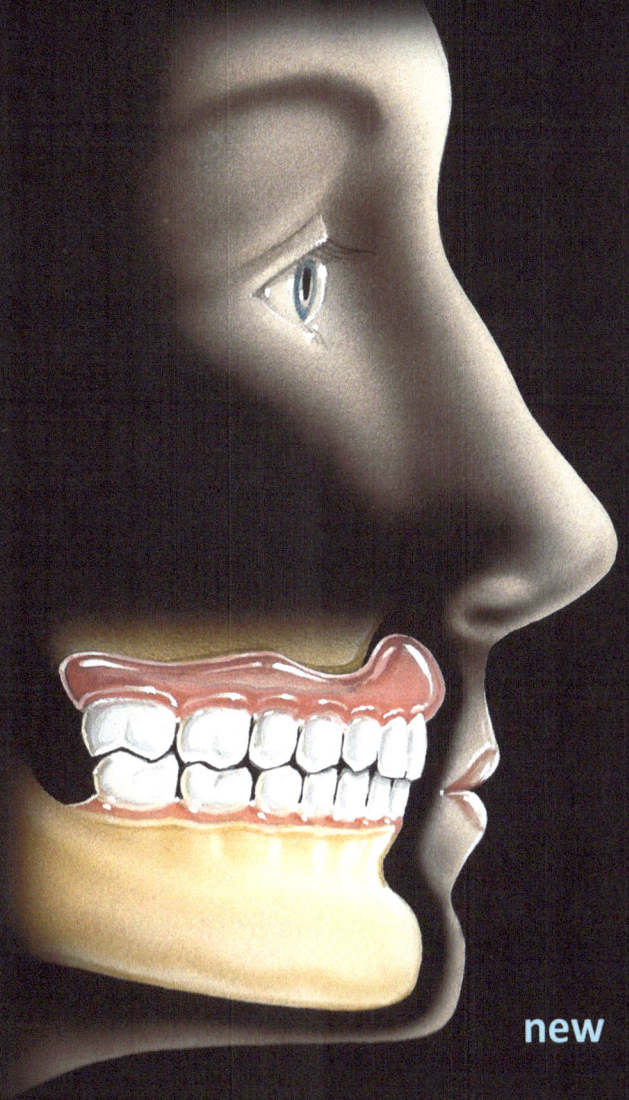

new

A properly fit denture can improve ones ability to chew food and improve digestion, avoid mouth sores, and improve ones facial features and profile.

Occlusion

Normal

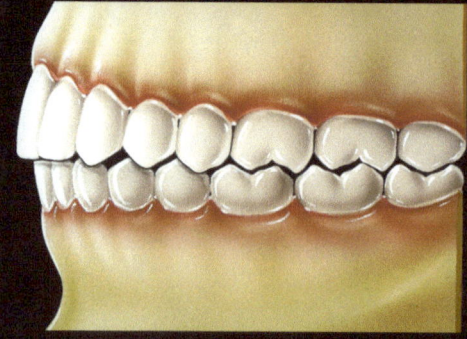

Class II

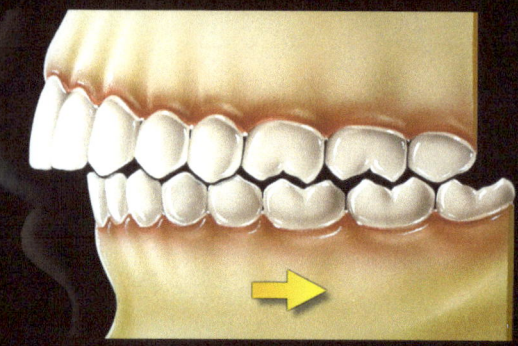

Class III

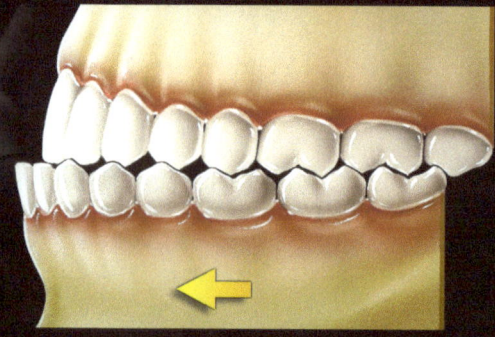

Occlusion refers to the biting alignment of the upper and lower teeth. Malocclussion refers to improper alignment. Class II malocclusion (overbite) is when the lower teeth are misaligned back from the normal position, and Class III malocclusion (underbite) describes when the lower teeth are misaligned forward.

www.ingramcontent.com/pod-product-compliance
Lightning Source LLC
Chambersburg PA
CBHW050834290526
45792CB00001B/393